7/08

ConsumerReports®
Guide to
Childproofing
& safety

Dedication

While writing the last chapter of this book, my biggest protector passed away, my mom, Sandra Schaefer. She was the ultimate guardian and defender and an inspiration to her children, grandchildren and everyone around her. She was always on the lookout for ways to safeguard her family—every question was important and no advice was too small. If she saw a toy or product recall on TV, she would call my siblings and me just in case we hadn't seen it. Any time there was a problem that could possibly affect my children, the phone would ring and it would be my mom. We all have that instinct to protect our children, but sometimes, instinct needs a little support. The advice and guidance of my mom was always in the back of my mind as I wrote this book. She taught me that a little extra knowledge can go a long way to keep a child safe. It can even save a life.

ConsumerReports®

Guide to
Childproofing
& Safety

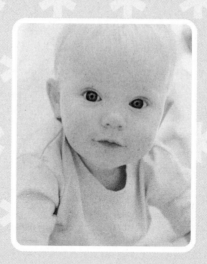

Jamie Schaefer-Wilson & the Editors of Consumer Reports

CONSUMERS UNION • YONKERS • NEW YORK

Consumer Reports Books

Editor, Books and Special Publications ....David Schiff
Author..Jamie Schaefer-Wilson
Contributing Editor..Susan Randol
Contributing Researcher..Maggie Keresey
Coordinating Editor ....Terese Christofferson
Copy Editor ....Alison France
Design Manager ....Rosemary Simmons
Contributing Art Director...Vicky Vaughn Shea
Illustrator ....Susan Yule Hunt
Associate Director, Content Resource Scheduling ....Nancy Crowfoot
Production Associate ....Terri Kazin
Technology Specialist ....Jennifer Dixon

Consumer Reports

Director, Editorial and Production Operations...................................David Fox
Design Director...George Arthur
Creative Director...Tim LaPalme
Product Manager, Publications Development ....Lesley Greene
Production Associate, Manufacturing and Distribution.............Mark Yatarola
Senior Director, Product Safety and
        Health Operations ....Carolyn Clifford-Ferrara
Program Leader ....Joan Muratore

Consumers Union

President...James Guest
Senior Vice President Information Products..............................John J. Sateja
Vice President and Editorial Director...Kevin McKean
Vice President and Technical Director ....Jeffrey Asher
Vice President, Publishing ....Jerry Steinbrink
Senior Director, Product Safety and Technical Public Policy ......Donald Mays

First Printing, May 2008

Copyright© 2008 by Consumers Union of United States, Inc., Yonkers, N.Y. 10703.

Published by Consumers Union of the United States, Inc., Yonkers, N.Y., 10703.

ISBN-13: 978-1-933524-17-7

ISBN-10: 1-933524-17-0

Manufactured in the United States of America

contents

About the Author

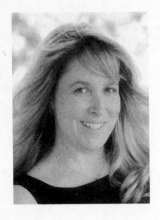

As an organizer for Consumers Union's Hazardous Imports Campaign, Jamie Schaefer-Wilson works to engage citizen activists in campaign activities and fights for tougher legislation for toys and other products.

She serves on several juvenile products committees for ASTM International, where she advocates for safer juvenile product standards. She has also worked as a consultant in Juvenile Product Testing and Safety for Consumer Reports. Jamie worked with the nonprofit Kids and Cars and is a certified child passenger safety technician. She is the author of *The Baby Rules: The Insider's Guide to Raising Your Parents*.

Jamie lives in New York with her husband, Steven Wilson, and their two daughters.

Introduction

We all love to see our children grow and explore, increasing their knowledge of and pleasure in the world around them. There's no greater pleasure in life than seeing your little one grow from tiny infant to a happy, healthy and independent young adult. Yet we know that the road to adulthood is filled with potholes that could harm our children, and we want to do all we can to steer them clear of the dangers.

When it comes to protecting our children, knowledge is power. And yes, there is so much to know that it can seem overwhelming, especially to new parents. The good news is that it's all pretty simple stuff. But even the simple stuff takes on new importance when the unexpected happens. That's why I've organized this book into short tips that are easy to read and digest. Some of the information you'll use every day—such as how to properly install a child car seat. Other information, I hope you'll never have to use—such as what to do if a child is burned.

Often it takes just one tidbit of information to prevent injury to a child or even save a young life. Of course it's impossible to predict emergencies and the only guarantee is that children are unpredictable and will constantly surprise you and keep you on your toes. So just start at Chapter One, take your time (as if you have any these days) and read through the book.

I urge you to share this book with your parents, baby sitters, friends, co-workers and anyone else who takes care of children. Armed with the knowledge that you are doing all you can to keep your kids safe, you'll have the peace of mind to focus on the great and all-too-brief pleasure of watching them grow.

Jamie Schaefer-Wilson

CHAPTER 1

The Nursery

Planning your nursery is one of the most exciting times in your life. You want to welcome your new arrival into just the right setting, one that reflects your love, your personality and your style. At the same time you want to select only the safest furnishings and furniture, and you want to arrange the room as safely as possible. So have a blast creating the room you want while following the safety tips in this chapter—when Junior is older, he's going to have his own opinions about the décor.

Paint in advance. Paint releases significant fumes for at least a week after it is applied. So, unless the nursery's new resident has an appointment for arrival, you'll want to have the room painted several weeks before your due date. If you had your heart set on blue or pink, you'll just have to compromise on another pastel. When you buy the paint, make sure it's marked for interior use and that it is a water-based latex paint, not alkyd. Also check the label to make sure the paint doesn't contain mercury.

Know about lead paint. If your house was built before 1978, there is probably lead in the paint on your walls. That's not a problem as long as the paint is in good shape and there is no chance it could chip or peel so that your child might eat it. If the paint is in good condition, you can paint over it. If there is a chance that the paint could chip or peel, you should have it tested for lead. If the results are positive, remove any deteriorating lead paint. For more information about lead in paint and what to do about it, see "Keeping the Lead Out," page 187.

Cut looped pull cords above the tassel and remove the equalizer buckle, if there is one. Then insert cord ends through tassels and knot the cord ends to keep tassels in place.

Let someone else paint. If you are pregnant, have someone else paint for you so you don't expose your fetus to any potentially harmful fumes. Ventilate the room with open windows and fans during and after painting.

Equalizer Buckle

Cut cord loops. The pull cords on some older window blinds and curtains have loops. They should be cut to eliminate the risk of strangulation. Place a cord tassel over each cut end and tie a knot to hold the tassel in place. If you are purchasing new window treatments for rooms where children will be, use cordless treatments.

Keep cords out of reach. Never place a crib or bassinet within reach of the cords for window blinds or curtains. Your baby could become entangled when you are not looking.

Hang nothing over the crib and changing table. Pictures, shelves or other items hanging over the crib or changing table could fall on your baby. And a child in a crib could easily pull something down as soon as she can pull herself to a standing position, usually at about 6 to 8 months.

Cut strings off wall hangings. Some have cords or strings that might entangle your child. Make sure any wall hangings like this are well out of your child's reach, or better yet, cut off the strings.

Install window guards. Even though you won't put the crib next to a window, it's a good idea to install window guards when you prepare the nursery. That way, you won't have to run out to the store the day your baby starts crawling, toddling, and before you know it, climbing. Get window guards that are screwed into the window frame. Don't get pressure-fit guards, which children can dislodge by pushing or leaning on them.

An insect screen will not prevent a child from falling through an open window. And you should have window guards whether you live in an apartment building or a house, and even if the nursery is on the first floor. They are sold in different sizes and adjust to various widths. Be sure they are tightly installed and have bars that are no more than

Window guards must be screwed securely into place.

4 inches apart and leave no gaps of more than 4 inches. Some guards have latches to allow for escape in case of emergency, and if this is the type you choose, make sure they're difficult for very young children to open.

Window stops work, too. As an alternative to window guards, you can purchase window stops to attach to the window frame. They prevent the window from opening more than 4 inches. Some new windows come with window stops already installed.

Keep furniture away from windows. An open window can become an even greater hazard when your toddler begins to climb onto things. So when you arrange the nursery, keep furniture away from windows. Also look out for stools or other small, light furniture that your toddler might be able to move to an open window. Stash them in a closet, on a high shelf when not in use.

Never purchase an antique or used crib or bassinet. It may be missing hardware that prevents it from collapsing or failing in some other way. Some older cribs have cutouts in the headboard or footboard. Whether old or new, your crib shouldn't have any cutouts or openings that could entrap your child's head, neck, arms, or legs.

Even if an old crib is in good shape, safety standards have improved over the years, so it's best to buy a new one if you can. A crib should be the one place you feel comfortable leaving your child alone.

Check the condition of the crib's paint. If your crib is painted, make sure the paint isn't chipped or peeling. This is especially important with older cribs that may have been coated with paint that contains lead— another reason not to use old cribs.

Check the crib for splinters. If you use an older crib, be sure to check it over thoroughly for cracks, splinters and rough edges, which could harm your baby.

Remove ribbons. If your bassinet has ribbons or bows make sure your child can't pull them off or become entangled. It's best to remove them or cut them shorter than 8 inches. If you decide to keep these decorative features, you need to be sure they are tightly fastened.

Check slat spacing. The slats in a crib or bassinet should be no farther apart than 2⅜ inches. If you can fit a can of soda through them, the opening is too large. You are more likely to find this problem in an older crib, but you can't be too safe when it comes to your baby, so check any crib you put him in. If you find you have purchased a crib that is unsafe, you should return it and report it to the Consumer Product Safety Commission (CPSC) at *www.cpsc.gov.*

Check corner posts. If your crib has corner posts or finial knobs they should stand at least 16 inches above the crib's end panels so that a child can't reach the top and get her pajamas caught. If the corner posts or finials are shorter than this, unscrew or saw them off so that the corners are no more than ¹⁄₁₆ of an inch higher than the crib ends or side panels. After sawing them off, you will need to sand the crib to eliminate splinters and sharp corners.

Inspect hotel cribs. When reserving a crib or a play yard at a hotel, try to find out the make and model number so you can check whether it has been recalled. Before you use either item, check thoroughly for loose screws or missing parts, and be sure the slats are no more than 2⅜ inches apart. Make sure the sheet is designed for the crib or the play yard, and is not a bed sheet that has been tucked underneath. Best bet: Bring your own crib sheet or play-yard sheet.

Check the hardware. Make it a habit to check the screws and bolts in your baby's crib to ensure nothing is loose, missing or damaged. Crib hardware can loosen over time and may need occasional tightening. If anything is missing or broken, contact the manufacturer for replacement parts.

Check mattress supports. Make sure that the system that supports the crib mattress isn't bent, broken or coming apart. Be sure it's secure and isn't in danger of falling. If the mattress is suspended on hangers attached to hooks on the end panels, check regularly to see that these are still connected. A handy time to look is when you are changing the crib sheet.

Make sure the mattress fits. Put your baby to sleep on her back on a firm mattress that fits tightly into the crib. There shouldn't be any cracks or openings between the crib and the mattress because a baby can get trapped in the smallest of spaces. A full-size crib has an interior surface of 28 inches by 52 inches. The mattress for a full-size crib should be 27¼ inches by 51⅝ inches, and no more than 6 inches thick. If you can place more than two fingers between the mattress and the crib frame, the fit isn't snug enough and there's a risk of head entrapment.

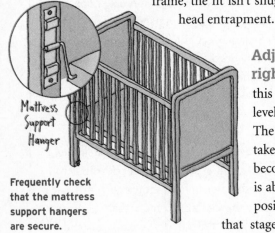

Mattress Support Hanger

Frequently check that the mattress support hangers are secure.

Adjust the mattress to the right height. Most cribs have this feature, some with only three levels and some with several levels. The higher levels make it easier to take your infant out of the crib but become dangerous when your child is able to pull herself to a standing position. Before your child reaches that stage—at around 6 months—the mattress should be at its lowest setting. Bumper pads and large toys help your little escape artist climb out, which is another reason they don't belong in the crib.

Let your baby sleep unencumbered. Don't wrap your bundle of joy in blankets or comforters when he's in the crib. He can quickly become entangled and might not be able to free himself. Pillows, quilts, comforters, sheepskins, stuffed animals or dolls don't belong in the bassinet or crib. And remember that babies can quickly overheat. Put yours to sleep in lightweight clothes and set the thermostat at a comfortable 70 degrees.

Use safe sleepwear. Infant sleepwear should fit snuggly and be made of flame-resistant fabric. There should be no drawstrings, ribbons or anything else that might catch on something. Buttons and snaps should be firmly attached to avoid becoming a choking hazard.

Remove the bottle. As your child gets older you may feel tempted to let him fall asleep with a bottle or sippy cup. Don't do this! Bottle nipples suffer from wear and tear over time and a small piece can break off and get caught in a baby's throat. Sleeping with a bottle or cup can also cause tooth decay and lead to ear infections.

Use the proper sheets. Use ones made to fit the mattress in your crib, bassinet or play yard. If a sheet isn't the correct fit, your baby may pull it up and become entangled. Test the sheet by pulling up on each corner to make sure it doesn't pop off the mattress corner.

Skip the crib gym. The safest crib is one that is free of gyms and other toys that stretch across the crib using strings, cords or ribbons. They can be dangerous for older or more active babies, and you have no way of knowing what your baby is doing in the middle of the night.

If you think you must use crib gyms or other crib toys, you can reduce the risks by following recommendations from the Consumer Product Safety Commission. Items should be free of points that your child's clothing could get caught on; they should be securely installed at both ends; they should be out of your child's reach; and they should be removed when your child is 5 months old or begins to push up on his hands and knees. Remove strings and cords from all toys and be sure there aren't any hanging into the crib or within reach of your baby.

Skip the bumpers, too. Crib bumpers are cute, but it's best not to use them. They need to be tied down with string, which is a potential hazard if not properly secured. If you do use a bumper, choose one that is thin, firm, and made of mesh, not one that is puffy or padded. It should fit around the entire crib and it should be secured in several places by ties or snaps. At a minimum, there should be a tie or strap at the top and bottom edges of each corner and in the middle of each long side. After tying the bumper to the crib, trim off excess string to prevent your baby from becoming entangled. The tie should be no longer than 8 inches.

Don't use a sleep positioner. Those wedge-shaped pieces of foam are designed to help babies sleep on their back. But the American Academy of Pediatrics says that none of these devices have been tested sufficiently to show that they are effective or safe.

Use the crib correctly. Don't lift your baby over the side of the crib without dropping the side first, or you'll be showing her how to escape. Also get in the habit of raising and locking the sides as soon as your baby is in the crib and check that all latches are locked.

Always put your baby to sleep on his back, not his stomach, to minimize the risk of sudden infant death syndrome (SIDS) and rebreathing, a sometimes fatal circumstance that can occur when a baby is sleeping on his stomach or trapped in soft bedding. As a result the child "rebreathes" his own carbon dioxide rather than breathing in oxygen-rich fresh air. The lack of oxygen can cause death.

Crib mobiles are for looking at, not for touching. They often have string or small attached pieces. Make sure your little one cannot reach the mobile so he can't become entangled or pull anything off. When he is able to push himself up on his hands and knees, the mobile should be removed from the crib.

Keep hanging objects out of reach. As with a crib, if you have a mobile or something else hanging over the changing table, be sure it doesn't hang low enough for your child to reach. Also, don't place your changing table next to curtain cords. A lot can happen when your attention and both hands are focused on changing your baby.

Never leave your child alone on a changing table. Although the table may seem low to you, for a child a fall from a changing table is like an adult falling from several stories and could be fatal. Keep everything you will need during changing within your reach. If you run out of diapers or forget your little one's outfit, carry her with you while you get what you need.

Don't rely on changing-table straps. Use them but be aware that they are only backup protection. They'll help keep your child in place, but the straps are no substitute for being there with your hand on your child at all times.

Remove oils and powders from your changing table. You may have received these in gift baskets or you may have bought them yourself thinking they were necessary for changing, but if your baby ingests or aspirates them it can be fatal.

Use furniture restraints. Fasten your changing table as well as any bookcases, armoires and dressers to walls with restraints that prevent tipping. Even seemingly stable furniture can become a tipping hazard—for example when a curious toddler opens all the drawers of a dresser. Also, you could accidentally tip a

Properly installed furniture straps prevent furniture from tipping onto your child.

furniture piece yourself. Some furniture comes with a strap or other means to fasten it to the wall. Or you can purchase a separate anti-tip fastener. In most cases you attach the anti-tip device to the furniture itself and then screw the unattached end into a stud in the wall. Follow the specific directions that came with the device.

Take care around gliders. A glider can be a great addition to your nursery, but it can also be a temptation for little ones who want to sit in it by themselves or figure out how this contraption works. As your child grows, you will need to teach her to keep her hands away from the gliding mechanism.

When your little explorer begins to climb, teach her not to use a glider, and especially the accompanying footstool, as a jungle gym. While the chairs themselves are not likely to tip over, you never know what someone young and ambitious can accomplish. The footstools are more prone to tipping.

Do not attach ribbon, string or yarn to a pacifier. They can become strangulation hazards.

CHAPTER 2

The Bathroom

As your little one starts crawling and exploring every nook and cranny of the house, discovers that food is just as much fun in his hair as in his mouth, and cake frosting makes a great face mask, you'll be spending plenty of cleanup time together in the bathroom. Some everyday items there can be attractive dangers to small children, so you'll need to put some thought into making the bathroom safe.

11

Have everything in reach. Bathing your newborn in a sink can be a bit nerve-racking at first. You're worried about keeping his head up, soap away from his eyes and water out of his mouth. Plus he's a bit squirmy and slippery. But don't worry: It gets easier, and you'll soon find yourself enjoying this wonderful time with your baby. In fact, as he grows and the bathroom becomes just another playroom, you might find yourself longing for those early, quiet baby baths.

Take your time and have everything at your fingertips, such as baby soap, shampoo, washcloth and towel. You don't want to find yourself reaching for anything. If you forget something like shampoo, skip it this time. He's not exactly playing in the dirt just yet.

Check the temperature. Before putting your little one in the bath dip your elbow in the water; it should be comfortably warm. Your elbow is more sensitive than your hand, so it will give you a better sense of whether the water temperature is in a good range for your baby's sensitive skin. Some baby bathtubs come with a temperature indicator, but some of these indicators are too slow, hard to read and difficult to use.

Test the waters first. If you turn on the faucet while bathing your baby or toddler, always make sure you test the water temperature before it touches your child. If you have a toddler who can sit on her own, you can use one hand to test the water while the other hand keeps her secure. You'll need two hands for a baby, so it's a good idea to keep a separate tub or other container of rinse water handy along with washcloths. This way, you won't have to turn on the faucet once your child is in the bath, and you can always keep one hand on your child.

Prevent scalding water. You can reduce the risk of a burn by setting your water heater at 120°F, or, if you live in an apartment building, ask the superintendent to do so. If the super can't help, you can purchase an anti-scald device that screws into place between the shower pipe and showerhead. The device senses water temperature and blocks the flow if the water becomes too hot. There are also anti-scald valves for the shower and tub that stop the flow by sensing water pressure changes. These are best for new construction, but a plumber can use them to replace existing valves.

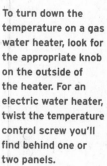

Stay vigilant! Allow nothing to distract you when you are bathing your child. The phone is ringing or someone is at the front door...what are you going to do? The answer is simple— nothing! It may seem safe enough to slip away for just a moment, especially as your child gets older and can sit up and play without assistance, but don't do it. It takes only a second for tragedy to occur when water is involved. Bath time can be as long or short as you like, but whether it's 5 minutes or 20, you need to be within arm's reach and forget about the outside world.

To turn down the temperature on a gas water heater, look for the appropriate knob on the outside of the heater. For an electric water heater, twist the temperature control screw you'll find behind one or two panels.

Make sure bath toys are safe and age-appropriate. Look for the manufacturer's age range on the front of the toy package. If it says it is not for a child under the age of 3, the product may have small parts that could break off. Even on toys labeled for young children, beware of small parts, such as eyes, that could be chewed, or suction cups that hold toys on the tub wall and are a choking hazard, or even toys that squeeze to a small enough size for a child to put in his mouth. In general, be sure that all toys are unbreakable and have no sharp parts. As all new parents quickly discover, infants try to put everything in their mouth, so to prevent a choking hazard, make sure the toys are too large to fit through the 1¾-inch diameter of a toilet-paper roll even when the toy is compressed.

Watch out for bath-set bags. If you have bath toys that came in a bag as part of a bath set, make sure the bag has a short handle. Some of these sets have been recalled because the handles are long enough to get wrapped around a child's neck.

Cups are great for bath-time fun. Bath toys are fun, but can take over your bath and they can break your bank. You'll need to change these toys often because they get filled with water and can become moldy. Sometimes something as simple as toy cups can be more fun than the most elaborate bath contraption. Give your child toy cups or durable drinking cups. Teach your child that, in the bath, these cups are for dumping water, not for drinking it. And don't use the plastic disposable kind, which can easily break into sharp pieces that can cut or choke your child.

Use washcloths instead of sponges. Either one will end up in your baby's mouth, but tiny pieces can easily break off sponges. And washcloths can go through a washer and dryer so they get really clean, while sponges have to air dry and can harbor harmful bacteria.

Do not use baby bath seats. You may feel the need to use one to help hold a slippery baby or to give a sense of security to a little one who is squeamish about bathing. But baby bath seats are not safety devices; in fact, they have been linked to about 120 drownings and 160 injuries since 1983. They can tip over, kids sometimes slip through the leg holes, and they often try to climb out or over the seat. The suction cups at the bottom of a baby bath seat must be attached to a smooth surface. If the tub is a slip-resistant or nonskid model, the suction cups will not adhere to the surface and the bath seat will slip. Even if the seat seems secured to the bottom or side of the tub, it can dislodge and tip, and can keep a helpless baby's face under water.

If you are looking for a more convenient and secure way to bathe your baby, consider getting a baby bathtub.

Use baby bathtubs with care. If you use one, be sure to keep at least one hand on your child, and everything within arm's reach, just as you would when bathing her in a sink or adult bathtub. Fill the tub with no more than 2 inches of water before you put the baby in it. Don't add more water while your baby is in it, and never put the baby bathtub into a larger tub that is filled with water because it can float around and tip. Place the baby bathtub on a flat, level surface that doesn't allow it to slip and makes it easy for you to handle your baby.

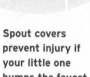

Spout covers prevent injury if your little one bumps the faucet.

Place a spout cover over the bathtub faucet. These soft covers can prevent injury if your child accidentally knocks his head on the spout. They also protect your child from a hot spout and sharp edges. Some spout covers are soft plastic in the shape of an animal. Others are inflatable plastic printed with a kid-friendly design.

Don't leave your baby with an older child. While siblings may love to bathe together, you must never leave a baby or toddler alone in the bath with another child. Even an older child might not be able to lift himself out of the bath, and he might not be able to lift a baby or younger child out of the bath if there's a problem.

Do not allow an older child who is out of the bath to supervise a younger child who is in the bath. The older one might not be able to help in an emergency, or be able to spot behavior that can lead to a dangerous situation in the bath. It takes an instant for a child to slip in the bath and end up with a mouthful of water. A baby or child can drown in less than 2 inches of water.

Always empty the tub as soon as bath time is over. It takes only a second for a curious infant, toddler or older child to go fishing for that bath toy and fall into the tub.

Be on hand for showers. At some point, usually around age 3 or 4, your little one will be ready to take a shower with your help and constant supervision. But first, be sure she can readily stand and move on her own in the shower without slipping. And don't toss out those bath toys yet, since she may still want a bath now and again.

By about 7 or 8, your child should be ready to shampoo her own hair, and wash and rinse herself. Even then, stay within arm's reach. She might slip, there could be a temperature surge, or she just may need your help in other ways. You might have to remove soap from her eyes or help her sidestep the shampoo that spilled on the floor.

Have a washcloth ready. Make sure your little one always takes a washcloth or small hand towel into the shower with her. She'll be prepared when soap inevitably gets in her eyes.

Place a slip-resistant mat in the shower stall or bathtub to give your little one (and the rest of the family, for that matter) more grip.

Lock up sharp items. Get in the habit of locking all razors, nail clippers, tweezers and other sharp objects in a cabinet with a childproof lock or latch. Before your child's bath or shower, make sure no one has absent-mindedly left a razor where a child can reach it.

Never dispose of razor blades, medicine, toothbrushes, small bottle caps or other potentially dangerous items in bathroom or bedroom wastebaskets. Once your child is crawling, he will naturally look into one, stick his hand in or tip it over. Use a wastebasket that he can't tip or reach into, and make sure it has a lid. If possible, put the wastebasket under the sink in a cabinet with a safety lock.

Dispose of Old Medications Properly

Flushing old medications down the toilet poses a danger to fish and wildlife. Instead, crush solid medications in a sealed plastic bag before tossing them into the trash. Combine liquid medications with sawdust or cat litter before sealing them in plastic bags and throwing them away.

Everyday items may actually be dangerous. Many products you keep in the bathroom will tempt a child. Some that seem harmless enough—mouthwash for example—are dangerous if ingested in large quantities. Even iron tablets or vitamin supplements containing iron can be dangerous in high doses. Keep vitamins, mouthwash, cleaning products, prescription and over-the-counter medicines, and bath oils and gels in the highest cabinets and install safety latches. You should check your cabinets regularly and dispose of outdated medicine.

Lock up your medication. Be sure your medicine is in child-resistant containers. Still, a determined child may be able to open them, so keep them in a locked cabinet. Never refer to medicine as "candy" or anything else that will tempt your child, even if you are trying to cajole Junior into taking his medicine. Also, never have a young child help you take medication.

Clearly label everything stored in your bathroom, including medicine, vitamins, hygiene products and cleaning supplies. But accidental ingestion can happen despite your precautions. If it does, you need to immediately know exactly what your child has taken.

Stash colorful soaps. Edible-looking soaps are confusing to a child. "Wash your mouth out with soap" can take a whole new meaning. If they're colorful or attractive to children, you need to keep them out of reach until you can teach your child that they are for cleaning and not for eating.

✳ The Bathroom

GFCI Guards Against Electrocution

Outlets with Ground Fault Circuit Interrupter (GFCI) protection are essential for a bathroom. If you have these outlets and accidentally drop your hairdryer or curling iron in water the circuit will be cut, preventing possible electrocution. Even with these outlets, try to avoid using any electrical equipment near water. You don't want to create a safety hazard.

The National Electrical Code requires GFCI protection on any outlets installed near sinks or tubs, or near potentially wet places like kitchen counters. If your house pre-dates the code requirement established in the early 1970s, it may not have this GFCI protection. But you can easily retrofit your outlets.

GFCI outlets have two buttons on them. One is labeled "TEST," the other

GFCI receptacles help prevent shocks in the bathroom.

"RESET." But if you don't have these outlets in your bathroom, don't run to the home center just yet. Your outlets might be protected by a GFCI circuit breaker (also identifiable by a "TEST" button) in your electric service panel. And one GFCI outlet can protect others farther down the same circuit, so if there are other GFCI outlets in you house, chances are the bathroom outlets are protected by one of them. To find out which outlets are protected by a given GFCI device, push the "TEST" button. If the bathroom outlets don't work until you hit the reset buttons, they are protected.

You should test and reset your GFCIs monthly to make sure they work. If a GFCI-protected outlet still has power when you press "TEST," replace the outlet or contact an electrician.

Keep the phone number for poison control handy. The Poison Control Center's toll-free phone number is 800-222-1212. The line is answered 24 hours a day and a representative will connect you to the nearest poison control center. Keep this number by all your phones so you will have it immediately on hand if you ever need it. You might want to tape the number to your phones so it won't get misplaced.

Put appliances away. Never leave your hair dryer, curling iron or other electrical appliance plugged in when you leave the bathroom. A curious toddler can turn on any of these appliances in a flash. And if an appliance falls into water while it is plugged in, it can electrocute a child who reaches for it, even if it is not turned on. If your child is in the bathroom with you, make sure she can't reach any electrical appliances that might get dropped or knocked into the sink, tub or toilet.

Install toilet latches on all toilet lids. As soon as a curious baby can pull himself up, he may decide to have a look inside the toilet or a toddler might try to fish out something he dropped in. In either case, he can go in headfirst if he loses his balance. The best toilet latches are easy for adults to use but hard for children, and they reset themselves after use.

Make sure your towel bars are securely fastened to the wall. Even if they are, remember that a towel bar is not a grab bar; it's designed to support the weight of a towel, not a person, even a little person. Try to hang your towels so your child can't reach up and pull on them. And as he grows, teach him that pulling the towel bar is a no-no. Likewise, be careful yourself not to whip towels off the bar when your child might be underneath.

Toilet-lid latches are essential when you have a baby or toddler in the house.

Buy bath mats and rugs with nonslip bottoms.
Many mats can act like banana peels when placed on slippery bathroom floors, a hazard for adults and children alike. Place a nonslip bathmat immediately in front of the shower stall or bathtub. People of any age

might sometimes have trouble finding their footing when exiting the bath or shower.

Stash the stool. You'll want a stool in the bathroom to help your toddler reach the sink faucet. But don't let him use the stool near a window where he might fall out, or near window cords that might strangle him. And be sure to stash the stool someplace where your child can't find it when you're not looking.

Child-proof the bathroom doorknob. Purchase a child-proof cover for the bathroom door knob that adults can open by gripping and turning the plastic cover. Kids won't be able to enter the bathroom alone.

CHAPTER 3

Your Toddler's Room

When your child outgrows his crib, it's time to transform the nursery into a toddler's bedroom. To make the transition a safe one, begin by looking at the room through the eyes of a 3-foot child who wants to open drawers and explore his domain the moment you leave the room. In this chapter you'll learn how to create an environment your mobile and curious toddler can safely enjoy exploring. To add to the fun, get your child involved in some of the decorating decisions. Remember though, that the latest trend quickly becomes old news and that children outgrow certain styles. Your daughter might think that Snow White is a decorating must now, but in a few months she'll prefer Sleeping Beauty, and in a year she'll want something totally different.

Create a new bed. When your child begins to climb out of the crib or reaches a height of 35 inches, it's time to leave the crib behind. Some children try to escape from the crib earlier than others, so be sure to make the switch if you see this behavior, even if your child is still less than 35 inches tall.

Use bed rails only with adult mattresses and box springs. Never install portable bed rails on a crib or toddler bed because the mattress is too small to support them. And don't use them on bunk beds, waterbeds, youth beds, inflatable mattresses, or a bed without a box spring. (Young children should never sleep on waterbeds.) Look for a certification sticker from the Juvenile Products Manufacturers Association (JPMA) on the rail or the packaging. Bed rails should be used when your child is about 2 until age 5.

A Look at Bed Options

There are different strategies to provide a safe bed for your child as he grows. One is to purchase a crib that converts to a toddler bed. Some even convert from a crib to a toddler bed and then to a full-sized bed.

The least expensive option is to go with a separate toddler's bed, one that is not part of a crib but rather a mini-version of a twin bed. Toddler beds are low to the ground and use a standard crib mattress. They have bed rails that are usually 2 inches above the top of the mattress. The rails are there to remind kids that they're getting close to the edge of the mattress, not to actually prevent them from falling out. A toddler's bed should suffice until your child outgrows it, usually at age 5 or around 50 pounds.

You might prefer getting a twin or full-sized bed and adding a portable bed rail to each side. Although this option is more expensive than buying a toddler's bed, it could conceivably work until your child leaves home. Transitioning from a crib is a major milestone for toddlers, and scary dreams are a fact of life for many youngsters, so it's nice to have a bed that can hold you, too, in case you need to comfort your child occasionally or read another bedtime story.

A bunk bed is also an option, but reserve the top bunk for children over the age of 6.

Follow the manufacturer's instructions when installing bed rails. If they leave a gap or loosen during the night, your child could get trapped, so use the rails strictly according to instructions and check them each night before use. Be sure they fit tightly with no gaps between the mattress and the rail, so that your child can't get stuck. Leave 9 inches between the bed rail and the footboard and headboard.

Don't use the wall as a bed rail. Putting a bed against the wall is not an acceptable substitute for a bed rail. Your child could get trapped between the wall and the mattress. Look for bed rails that can be securely attached on each side of your child's bed.

Bed rails must be installed tightly against the bed, with a 9-inch space between them and the headboard and footboard.

Take care with bunk beds. If you choose a bunk bed for your child, note that thousands of injuries occur each year from children falling from the top bunk. While many of these injuries are minor, a fall from a top bunk can have disastrous results. Don't let a child less than 6 years old sleep on the upper bunk. If your bunk bed can be made into two separate beds, use it in this configuration or store one bunk until your children are ready to use it safely.

No protrusions allowed. Make sure nothing extends more than $\frac{3}{16}$ of an inch from your bunk beds. This includes the corner posts of the bed, any unusual configuration of the top rail, and the ladder. A child can hang himself on a protrusion. Never hang anything on a bunk bed either, such as a belt or jump rope.

Guardrails should be
securely installed at
the proper height to
ensure that the top
bunk bed is safe.

Make sure bunk-bed guardrails are secure.

They can fail, causing a child to fall to the floor. Make sure you have guardrails on all sides and that they are firmly attached with screws or bolts. Check often to make sure the fasteners remain tight. Guardrails should extend at least 5 inches above the mattress. There should be no more than 3½ inches of vertical space between them and the bed frame.

Post protrudes
no more
than ³⁄₁₆"

5"

No more
than 3½"

Guardrails
firmly attached

Watch for gaps.

While the bed might seem secure against a wall, your child can become trapped between it and the bed or fall through gaps that form between them. Use guardrails on both sides of the upper and lower bunks.

Only the correct size mattress only.

Bunk beds and mattresses come in two lengths—regular and extra long, with extra long being 5 inches longer than regular. Using a regular-length mattress on an extra-long bed creates a gap that is a strangulation hazard.

Make sure you have cross ties.

The mattress foundation on some bunk beds merely rests on small ledges attached to the bed frame. This is dangerous because an upper-bunk mattress can become dislodged when a child pushes on it from underneath, causing it to fall on the child on the lower mattress. Make sure your upper-bunk foundation rests on cross ties to prevent it from falling. The cross ties can be metal straps, wooden slats, or wire. Make sure they are securely attached to the bunk-bed structure.

Secure the ladder. If your bunk bed comes with a ladder, be sure it is securely attached to the bed frame and can't move when your child climbs up and down. Check for missing or loose ladder rungs and replace them immediately.

Labels: Foundation, Mattress, Wood Slat, Metal Strap, Cross Wire

Use a baby monitor again. When your child first moves to a big bed, dust off the baby monitor and keep it in his room for the first few weeks. You might want to use it longer than that if he is the adventurous type. You'll want to know if he has gotten out of bed when he's supposed to be sleeping.

Cross ties prevent the top mattress from falling on a child in the lower bunk.

Buy flame-retardant sleepwear, and be sure your child never goes to bed wearing necklaces or other jewelry that can become a strangulation hazard. Your child's sleepwear must be either flame retardant or tight fitting. Don't allow her to sleep in loose-fitting or oversized garments such as T-shirts, sweatshirts, or other apparel made from fabrics that aren't flame-resistant. Those garments ignite more easily. Also make sure there are no drawstrings, especially around the neck area, and no loose buttons, snaps, bows, etc. that could pose a choking hazard, since a toddler still puts things in his mouth.

Add a night-light to your child's room and to the hallway outside his room. While you don't want to encourage him to leave his room in the middle of the night, he may find himself in the hallway looking for you. To be sure the night-light meets safety standards, look for safety symbols from UL (Underwriters Laboratories), Canadian Standards Association (CSA), or Electrical Testing Laboratories (ETL).

Make a nighttime plan. Tell your child what he should do if he gets scared in the middle of the night and thinks he needs you. Should he stay in his room and call for you? Or do you feel comfortable letting him find his way to your room? Even if you have instructed him to stay put, make sure the path between your room and his is well-lighted in case he "forgets." When your child is potty-trained and can safely go to the bathroom by himself, make sure that he can find the closest one at night and that the path is illuminated.

Use gates—again. If your child's bedroom is near a staircase, consider adding a gate to prevent her from tumbling down the stairs in the middle of the night. If the gate is at the top of the stairs, it should be mounted with hardware; if it's in the child's doorway, it can be pressure-mounted. The gate can be a temporary measure until she gets used to her bed and her room.

An emergency key makes it easier to rescue a locked-in child.

Think ahead about door locks. It's bound to happen—one day your young child will accidentally lock himself into his bedroom or the bathroom. So be prepared with an emergency door key—a two-pronged, easy-to-grip opener that works on both push and turn locks. You should be able to find one at your local hardware store, or search for "emergency door key" at online sources.

Prevent pinched fingers. As your little one begins opening and closing doors, you'll want to be sure he can't catch his fingers. This requires two types of devices: a panel that screws into the door frame to cover the hinge side, and a pinch-guard bumper that fits on the latch edge of the door to prevent it from closing all the way. You'll need to remove this device from bedroom doors at night for fire safety. (See "Sleep with Bedroom Doors Closed," page 178.) You can find both of these devices for sale online.

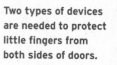

Install window guards. If your child's room doesn't already have window guards or window stops, be sure to install them before he makes the transition from crib to bed. Even if a window doesn't seem accessible, it could be; your child is now capable of pushing furniture over to the window and climbing. Even the bathroom should have a window guard, since your child soon will begin using that room alone. He can easily move a bathroom stool to a window for a better look outside or climb on the toilet if it is near a window. Teach your child not to push or lean on window guards. Check the screws regularly to make sure the window guards are securely fastened. Remember, a screen will not prevent a child from falling through a window. (See "Install window guards," page 3, and "Window stops work, too," page 4.)

Two types of devices are needed to protect little fingers from both sides of doors.

Make sure window cords are safe. If the windows in your child's room have blinds or curtains with pull cords, make sure the cords don't have loops, which are a strangulation hazard. (See "Cut cord loops," page 2 to learn how to make them safe.)

Don't touch that lamp! Teach your child to keep away from lamps. You should be in charge of turning lamps off and on, not your child.

Check that any lamp in your child's room has a UL, ETL, or CSA sticker indicating that it meets current safety standards.

Keep cords out of reach. A child can easily pull down a lamp by the cord. Wrap it and secure it.

Keep outlets covered. Just because your child is no longer crawling around on her hands and knees doesn't mean that outlets are no longer a hazard. In fact, she'll probably notice the outlets more and have easier access to things she can try to stick into them.

Don't put coveted items out of reach in your child's room. She's probably curious about the items on the upper shelves in her closet, but don't tempt fate. Keep the items she's allowed to have within arm's reach. If she can't have something or it isn't appropriate for her age, remove it from her room rather than storing it in her closet.

Use anti-tip devices and drawer latches. Attach your children's furniture—such as the dresser—securely to the wall with these devices. (See "Use furniture restraints," page 9.) Also add safety latches to dresser drawers to prevent your child from opening the drawers, climbing on them, or pulling a drawer completely out onto himself. (See "A Look at Childproof Latches and Locks," page 36.)

Use the lower shelves on your child's bookcase. Your child will want to explore her environment. So if you have bookshelves or a bookcase in her room, store the items she will want on a lower shelf. Storing items on higher shelves won't deter her; she will eventually try to reach them.

Nix the TV. You don't need another electrical hazard in your toddler's bedroom. And you won't have to worry about it falling off its stand or shelf and hurting your child.

CHAPTER 4

The Kitchen

Your kitchen is more than a place to cook—it's a room where family and friends gather to catch up on the day, grab a snack, or enjoy informal meals. But there can be more potential hazards in the kitchen than in any other room in the house. Like the bathroom, the kitchen has water, electricity and potentially dangerous chemicals, such as cleaning products. It also has fire or other sources of heat, another possible hazard. Top it off with drawers full of sharp objects, and you have plenty of risks for your little ones. But if you follow the simple precautions in this chapter, you can welcome the whole family into the kitchen with peace of mind.

Keep a fire extinguisher handy. A multipurpose dry-chemical one is best. Cooking is one of the most common causes of home fires, and burning grease, oil or fat is the most common type of kitchen fire. Throwing water on a grease fire can cause the grease to splatter, spreading the fire.

If there's an oven or microwave fire shut the door and keep it shut. Turn off the power and, if possible, unplug the appliance. Call 911 immediately and grab your fire extinguisher. If the fire spreads or grows while you're waiting for help to arrive, stand back a few feet and discharge the fire extinguisher at the base of the fire.

Stay in the kitchen. Cooking was the leading cause of fire and injuries caused by fire in structures in 2005, the most recent year that the U.S. government gathered statistics. Never leave the kitchen while food is cooking. It may seem tedious to stay in the room waiting for water to boil or pasta sauce to simmer, but that is the best way to avoid a serious kitchen fire.

What to Do if Your Child Is Burned

If your child is burned, first and foremost, you must try to stay calm. The more nervous you are, the more upset your child will become. You need a level head to soothe him and to get medical help as soon as possible if he needs it. Here's what else you need to do:

- Immediately flush the burn with cool water to reduce skin temperature, and keep cool water running over it. Do not use ice because it can make the burn worse by decreasing blood to the area.

- If the burn is to an arm or leg, elevate it to reduce swelling.
- If the burn blisters or is larger than a quarter, call your doctor immediately.
- If your child, or anyone else, is burned around the head, there is danger of airway injury. Take her to the hospital immediately if you see burns to the face, singed nasal hairs or burns around the mouth. In this case always keep the child's head elevated.
- Don't take a chance with any burn. If you have any doubts, take your child to the hospital immediately.

Remove stove knobs. The easiest way to make sure your child can't turn on the stove when you're not looking is to remove the knobs when the stove is not in use. An alternative is to purchase stove-knob covers. Leave these covers off or open (some models have hinges) when cooking so you can quickly turn off burners in an emergency. If you are buying a new stove, consider one with knobs on the top where your child can't reach them. Even with stovetop knobs you need to remain vigilant; a child could pull a chair over to the stove to reach them.

Use the back burners. You could install a stove guard, a transparent piece of plastic that you place across the front of the stovetop to keep your child from reaching pots and pans. But these guards make it awkward to use the stove. An easier solution is to get in the habit of using the back burners. If you need the front burners too, turn the handles of pots and pans sideways so they don't hang over the front of the stove. In fact, turning the handles when using the back burners is also a good habit; it will make pots and pans that much more difficult for growing children to reach.

Even a cold stove can be dangerous. A stove may seem benign when it's off, but there are more hazards than meet the eye. Keep your child away from the stove whether it is hot or cold, on or off. Don't allow your kids, or anyone else for that matter, to put their weight on an open stove door. The door could become a lever, causing the stove to tip over.

Cooking on the back burners helps keep pots out of your child's reach.

Anti-tip brackets are a must for stoves. Since 1991, voluntary safety standards have required stoves to be

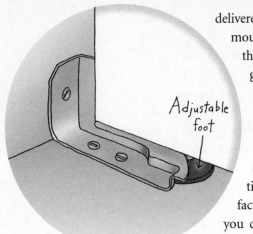

Adjustable foot

Anti-tip devices prevent the stove from tipping onto your child.

delivered with metal anti-tip brackets and mounting hardware. But don't assume the installer used them. To check, grab the back of the stove and try to tip it up slightly.

If your stove doesn't have brackets, ask the manufacturer for a tip restraint so you can attach it yourself. It's best to use a tip restraint designed by the manufacturer for your specific stove, but if you can't get one from the manufacturer, you can buy one from your local home center or hardware store. The brackets are usually designed to be screwed to the floor or into a wooden baseboard or the wall framing behind the stove (not just into drywall or plaster). The bracket captures one of the stove's rear feet.

Utensils are not toys. Kids love to play with kitchen utensils, but letting them do this is not a good idea. They'll be more likely to reach for a pot of boiling water on the stove if it's the same pot they had fun playing with on the floor yesterday. So don't use pots and pans or any kitchen utensils as toys. Instead, keep an activity box filled with crayons, coloring books, stickers, or other items to occupy your child while you cook. Bring it into the kitchen with you each time; don't leave it on the counter, where it might encourage climbing.

An empty dishwasher can injure. Common sense tells you to keep children away from an open dishwasher filled with knives and forks. But an open dishwasher is dangerous to small children even when empty. A dishwasher rack is basically a series of blunt spikes. If you child falls onto a rack, he will almost certainly land face first and could be seriously

Putting Out a Pan Fire

The first step is prevention. Never leave cooking unattended on the stove, clean up grease spills right away, and keep a pan lid and oven mitt handy. If a pan does catch fire, here's what to do:

1. If the fire is already spreading, leave the house. Close the door behind you and call 911.
2. If the fire is still only in the pan, put on your oven mitt and smother the flames by sliding the lid over the pan. Keep the lid on until the pan is completely cool.
3. Turn off the burner—but only if you can do so without getting your hands, arms, clothing, body or hair anywhere near flames, smoke or the hot pan.
4. Never pour water on a grease fire. The water will boil intensely, causing burning liquid to spew onto everything nearby.
5. DO NOT try to move the pan to the sink or other location. The flames can sweep back over the pan handle, burning you or setting fire to your hair or clothes.
6. If you don't have a lid at hand, or if it fails to extinguish the fire, use your fire extinguisher. But stand back a few feet from the pan—the force of the spray may push burning liquid out of the pan—and sweep the nozzle back and forth at the base of the fire.

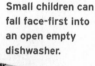

injured. So don't ask a small child to help load or unload the dishwasher. It's best if she is out of the kitchen while you do this chore.

Small children can fall face-first into an open empty dishwasher.

Don't store cleaners under the sink. Keep them in a high cabinet with a childproof lock or latch separate from food and away from curious kids. Unfortunately the hazard is increased because some liquid cleaners are colorful and, worse, packaged in containers that look quite similar to those used for fruit drinks.

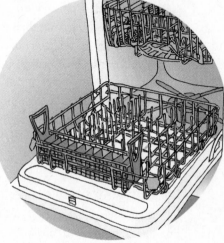

Lock up all cleaning products. Many of them can cause severe injuries, such as chemical burns or even death. In addition to keeping cleaning products in a locked cabinet, make sure containers are securely closed, and be sure to clean up any spills immediately.

Keep cleaning products in original, labeled bottles. Don't pour them into smaller bottles to disperse where you'll use them around the house. If your child ingests a cleaning product, you must immediately know what it is. And more bottles means more opportunities for your child to get her hands on them. If anything is missing a label, throw it out.

Take out only the products you will use at the moment. That way there is less chance you will inadvertently leave a dangerous item out where your child can get it.

Lock up matches. If you store your matches in the kitchen be sure to keep them locked in a cabinet well out of your child's reach.

Dispose of plastic wrappers and bags. Most of what we buy in the grocery store is wrapped in plastic, and we often carry it all home in plastic bags. Babies and toddlers will put anything in their mouth, and they love to put things over their heads. So throw away all plastic wrappers and plastic bags immediately in a garbage pail with a latch to reduce the risk of suffocation and airway obstruction.

Stow wrap boxes. If you purchase plastic wrap, aluminum foil or wax paper in boxes that have a sharp edge for cutting, be sure to keep them out of your toddler's reach. A small child can easily open them and cut himself on the sharp edges.

Lock up your trash. Sooner or later your child will become fascinated by the garbage pail. She may just want to throw things in as she sees you do. That's more of a nuisance than a hazard (like when she decides

Mommy doesn't need her watch anymore). The real danger begins when she wants to take things out of the trash and may be surprised by things like sharp metal lids. Keep the garbage pail in a locked cabinet or add a childproof latch to a covered pail.

Use caution when handling hot food or drinks. Never carry hot food or liquids and your baby at the same time. Allow food to cool before serving it to children.

Unplug your kitchen appliances when not in use. This will prevent a curious toddler from turning on appliances if he gets a notion to play chef. And whether they're on or off, keep appliances, cords and plugs out of your child's reach so he can't pull them off the counter.

Carriers or bouncers belong on the floor. With a newborn, your first instinct may be to bring your infant carrier or bouncer into the kitchen and to place it at eye level. While it may seem that you can better supervise your infant at a higher level, always place the carrier or bouncer on the floor, never on a countertop, a table, or a chair, where there is the potential for it to fall. Make sure the carrier isn't tilted so far forward that your infant's head falls onto her chest, which could obstruct breathing. And never carry a bouncer with your child in it; the toy bar is not intended for use as a carrying handle.

Keep walkers out of the kitchen. Walkers are unsafe, according to the American Academy of Pediatrics. If you insist on using one, at least keep it out of the kitchen. There are too many opportunities for her to scoot into trouble. She could bump into the hot stove or oven. Or she might reach that sharp item you are using. You might not notice her scoot behind you just as you step back. If your kitchen is big enough you can put your child in a stationary activity center while you cook, as long as she can't reach the stove. (See "Walkers can increase your baby's exposure to hazards," page 61.)

Although child-proof latches and locks are no substitute for your own vigilance, they are the most effective ways to keep young children out of large kitchen appliances as well as cabinets in the kitchen, bath, garage, or anywhere else you keep potentially dangerous items. Here is a look at some of the most popular types.

Type	Applications
Cabinet or drawer locks (push-type)	Most are screwed inside a drawer or cabinet, although some come with an adhesive strip that can be used for installation.
Cabinet or drawer locks with swivel or disable feature	Has a swivel feature or disable option to allow temporary disarming. Most must be screwed inside drawer or cabinet, although some come with an adhesive strip that can be used for installation.
Revolving-cabinet locks, also called lazy-Susan locks	Prevents a child from opening the revolving door on an L-shaped corner cabinet.
Magnetic cabinet/ drawer locks	A magnetic "key" unlocks the latches on your drawers or cabinet doors.
Sliding cabinet locks	Will only work on cabinets with side-by-side/ double doors, with knobs or loop handles. You slide the catch to the proper length for the spacing of your cabinet door handles.
Stove-knob covers	Hinged covers go over stove knobs to prevent children from turning them. Disk type goes under stove knobs to lock them in the "off" position.
Appliance locks	This is usually a strap with a buckle that prevents a child from opening a fridge, oven, microwave, etc. Some are latches with a catch that can be disabled when kids aren't around.
Oven locks	This is typically attached to the inside of the oven to keep a child from opening the door.

Pros	Cons
Out of sight, so a child may have less chance to see how they work. Can be used on single-door cabinets, unlike sliding cabinet locks.	May require a drill and screwdriver to install.
Grandparents can install these and "arm" them only when the grandkids visit. Can be used on single-door cabinets, unlike "sliding" cabinet locks.	You must remember to reconnect the latches. May require a drill and screwdriver to install.
One lock prevents opening both sides of the cabinet.	
With an inside-mounted lock, nothing shows on the outside of the drawer or cabinet. Can be used on single-door cabinets, unlike "sliding" cabinet locks.	Not easy to install. And if you misplace the "key," you have a problem!
Not a permanent installation, so it's easy to remove when not needed.	Prominently visible. And you must remember to put the lock back in place.
Prevents a child from turning oven or stove burners on. Works on gas grills, too.	Removing the knobs and putting them out of a child's reach accomplishes the same thing.
	The latch/catch type can be easy enough for a child to open.
Keeps a child out of the oven.	

Dry pet food is a choking hazard. Until your child is old enough to learn that this food is for Fido, not for him, you'll need keep him away from this not-so-tasty treat. Try to feed your pet out of your child's reach and remove the dish as soon as it is done eating.

Make sure you have GFCI protection. Electrical outlets with Ground Fault Circuit Interrupter (GFCI) protection are essential for a kitchen. If an appliance that's plugged into a GFCI-protected outlet falls into a sink full of water, power to the circuit will be cut off, preventing possible electrocution. Even with these outlets, try to avoid using any electrical equipment near water—you don't want to count on the device completely. (See "GFCI Guards Against Electrocution," page 18.)

Discourage climbing in the kitchen. If something will attract little kids, don't store it over the stove or leave it on the counter, because you don't want to encourage them to reach for it. In addition, these extra items can get in your way, causing a fire hazard around the stove. You or a child might knock something onto a lighted burner as you juggle cooking while watching a kid or three.

CHAPTER 5

Food and Dining

Feeding your baby might seem like the easiest thing to do safely, and in the beginning it can be. During the first few months your biggest worry may be grabbing the wrong thing out of the fridge at 2 a.m. when you feel like you are walking in your sleep. As you'll discover in this chapter, once your child moves on to pureed vegetables and fruits you'll need to watch out for allergies as well as some seemingly harmless items that could be choking hazards. And as she begins to toddle, you'll need to be alert to the furniture safety tips in this chapter as well. But before you dig into this safety advice, here is a fun tip: Be sure to have a camera handy when you offer your child a new food. You'll want to catch the reaction, whether it's a screwed-up face that says "Yuck!" or an expression of delight that says "Yum!"

If you plan to use a breast pump, buy a new one. To prevent the spread of viruses or bacteria, don't borrow or share with another mother. Milk can be sucked into the pumping mechanism, which, in most pumps, can't be sterilized or even thoroughly cleaned. Some pumps can be reused for another child of the same mother because they have a barrier to prevent contamination of the pumping mechanism. Many pumps don't have this barrier, so check with the manufacturer before using with baby number two. If you do keep the pump for future babies, be sure to clean it as thoroughly as you can before putting it away. If you have doubts about cleanliness, get a new pump.

Check the bottle nipples for wear and tear before each use to make sure they aren't cracked or brittle. Replace any nipples that seem worn and routinely replace them every three months. Your baby could choke if a piece of nipple breaks off in his mouth.

Use the right bottle-nipple size. They come in different sizes and are also made for different age ranges, so check the package. The size of the nipple hole varies too, so formula or milk can be released at different rates. Follow the age recommendations, but you'll still need to be attentive. If your baby begins to choke or gag during feeding, he may not be ready to graduate to the next size just yet.

Watch your caffeine and alcohol intake if you are breast-feeding. In general, a cup of coffee or tea or a glass of cola is fine, and one alcoholic drink a day or less has not been shown to be harmful. But if your baby is fussy or won't go to sleep, you might want to try reducing your caffeine intake. Keep in mind that coffee, tea and cola are not the only sources of caffeine; it's found in chocolate and in foods flavored with coffee and chocolate. Plus, caffeine is an ingredient in some medicines, particularly over-the-counter pain relievers, cold medicines and appetite suppressants. If you are nursing, be sure to ask your doctor about diet restrictions.

Follow storage limits for breast milk. You can store it for up to three months in a freezer that has a separate door. If you have a freezer compartment inside a refrigerator, it should be stored there for no more than two weeks, because refrigerator doors are opened and closed more frequently than freezers. If your refrigerator is kept between 32° to 39° F., you can keep breast milk there for up to eight days. In any case, there isn't a completely failsafe way to store milk in the refrigerator. Your fridge could go on the fritz or may not operate at the ideal temperature range. Always smell the milk before you give it to your baby to be sure it is still good.

Record storage dates. If you freeze your breast milk be sure to label the bottle with the date you stored it to prevent using milk that's too old. And of course you should always use the oldest milk first. It's also a good idea to keep a record of the foods you eat each day in case your baby has a bad reaction to your milk.

Ensure that formula is fresh. Mix formula just before you use it instead of storing premixed formula in the fridge. Check the date on the cans or labels. This use-by date, required by the Food and Drug Administration, indicates that the manufacturer guarantees the nutrient content and quality up to then. Never use formula past this date for nutritional reasons, as well as quality. Wash the lids before you open them.

Discard leftover milk or formula. Breast milk can be kept at room temperature (66° to 72°F.) for up to 2 hours. If your baby doesn't finish his bottle, don't put the milk or formula back in the refrigerator for later use. Whatever is left over must be thrown away.

Don't microwave milk or formula. If you refrigerate breast milk or formula that comes premade, you will need to warm it before use. But don't heat it in the microwave, because it can cause hot spots in the liquid that can cause serious burns. Tried-and-true methods are best: Just run warm water over the bottle or set it into a bowl of warm running water.

Shake after heating. You don't want your breast milk or formula to overheat, so be sure to run it under water that is warm, not hot. Then gently swirl it to disperse the heat and test the bottle by pouring a few drops onto your wrist. Don't shake the bottle too hard or too much; you want to disperse the heat without creating air bubbles.

Boil water for formula. Use either tap or bottled water to mix powdered or liquid formula. Boil the water for one minute, and then let it cool before mixing. You can skip the boiling if you use sterile bottled water.

Never prop the bottle. No matter how exhausted you might feel at that 3 a.m. feeding, never prop up your baby's bottle—always hold it yourself. Propping can cause your baby to choke. Only by holding the bottle yourself can you remove it quickly enough if your baby gags because he needs air or because the formula or milk is flowing too quickly.

As your child gets older and begins to hold the bottle, don't try to make it easier for her by propping the bottle on something. She will have to hold it up herself because no matter how old your child is, a propped bottle can lead to choking.

Never prop your baby's bottle. Keep an eye on your baby to make sure he isn't struggling, and tilt the bottle up slightly to reduce the chance of air bubbles.

Don't take your baby to bed with you. It is so tempting to take that sweet little baby into your bed after a nighttime feeding or to calm him if he is crying, but don't do it. Every year babies suffocate in bed because an adult rolled onto them, they got caught in the bedding, or got wedged between the mattress and another object or strangled in rails or openings in the bed. Even if your intention is just to enjoy your infant in bed for a bit while you are awake, don't take the chance—you could easily fall asleep. After feeding, put your baby back in his crib or bassinet with its proper mattress that is free of suffocation hazards. (See "Make sure the mattress fits," page 6.)

Check with your doctor before starting solid foods. Most babies are ready to start solid food, such as iron-fortified cereal, when they are 6 months old, pureed fruits and vegetables at 6 to 8 months and pureed meats around 8 months old. But check with your pediatrician before beginning solid foods to get food recommendations. Continue breastfeeding or formula for the first year. Your baby should reach certain developmental milestones before starting solid foods. He should be able to:
* Sit up unsupported.
* Display good control of his head and neck.
* Show an interest in eating by opening his mouth when a spoon is presented to him.
* Keep some food in his mouth.

Consider family history. If one or both parents have any type of allergy follow these guidelines, after checking with your pediatrician:
* No cow milk until age 1. (This applies to all babies, not just ones with a family history of allergies.)
* No eggs until age 2.
* No peanuts, tree nuts, fish or shellfish until age 3.

A peanut allergy requires special care. It can cause anaphylaxis, a life-threatening condition that can restrict breathing, cause a drop in blood pressure, and loss of consciousness. It takes vigilance to create a peanut-free environment for a child who is allergic to them, especially because people with peanut allergies should also avoid tree nuts. Food products sold in bakeries and ice-cream shops often come in contact with peanuts, for example. Read ingredient labels thoroughly as you shop. You might find tree nuts in cereal, crackers, barbecue sauces and ice cream. Also look for label warnings about food that may have been made on machines that were also used to make products containing peanuts. Chocolate candy bars are a common example.

Never give honey to your baby. It can cause a type of botulism in a baby. You may have heard of parents putting honey on a pacifier to calm a baby or to get him to suck. Until your child is 1 year old, do not give him honey or add it to his food, water or formula.

Watch for These Food-Allergy Symptoms

When your doctor gives you the green light to start your baby on solid foods, she'll recommend food groups for you to add one at a time every four or five days. This will help you identify foods to which your baby might be allergic. The foods that most often cause allergic reactions in children are eggs, milk, peanuts, soy and wheat. Children usually will outgrow an allergy to eggs, milk, soy and wheat, but not to peanuts, tree nuts, fish or shrimp.

Here are some food-allergy symptoms to watch for. They can typically arise anytime between a few minutes to two hours after eating the food:
• Wheezing or difficulty breathing
• Vomiting
• Diarrhea
• Skin rashes or hives. A hive can appear anywhere on the body in groups or singly. They are red- or skin-colored welts, often itchy, with clearly defined edges. They can go away in minutes or remain for hours.
• Tingling, burning or itchy tongue. (Your baby may rub her tongue.)
• Swelling of the lips, tongue or throat, resulting in breathing difficulty.
• Abdominal cramps. Your baby might hold her stomach, pull her legs up or cry in a way that indicates pain.
• Drop in blood pressure. Your baby or child will become pale and light-headed and might faint.

If your child exhibits any of these symptoms besides rashes or hives, call 911 immediately. If she has hives or a rash, call your pediatrician to ask for guidance. Do this even if your child has had a rash or hives in the past, and even if you already have an antihistamine prescription that has worked before. You want to determine the cause of the allergy.

When heating baby food, stir it well before giving it to your little one. This is especially important if you use a microwave oven, which heats food unevenly. Taste the food to test its temperature before serving.

Never feed your baby with a disposable plastic spoon. They can break in your baby's mouth and lead to injury or choking. It's best to use spoons designed for babies. They aren't prone to breaking and many are coated so they won't conduct heat like a metal spoon. You can find baby spoons in the baby-food section of most supermarkets and stores that sell juvenile products. Keep an extra in your diaper bag so you won't be caught without one.

Take care with small foods. Your pediatrician will tell you when it's time to start giving your baby finger food, such as small pieces of soft cheese, and well-cooked turkey or well-cooked pasta. But you still need to avoid anything small that might be a choking hazard, including grapes, hot dogs, popcorn, nuts, raisins, grape or cherry tomatoes, uncooked sliced vegetables or fruits, such as carrots or apples. Also avoid hard candy, chewy or sticky candy, gum, clumps of peanut butter, or chunks of meat or cheese. You should avoid these foods until your child is about 4 years old. After that, make sure she eats slowly and thoroughly chews her food. Even after age 4, it's a good idea to cut grapes and other round foods.

Remove pits and seeds. Small children can choke on them, so remove them before serving fruits or vegetables.

Teach good eating habits. Active older kids often like to chow down quickly so they can get back to whatever they were doing before mealtime. It may take seemingly endless reminding, but it's important to get them into the habit of eating one piece of food at a time and chewing it thoroughly. Teach them that food is to be eaten at the table and not while playing, running, or even walking.

Eat, then talk. Of course you want meals to be a time for enjoyable conversation. But choking can happen if kids are talking or laughing while eating. Teach your child that whatever is on her mind can be said once she swallows the food in her mouth.

Don't force eating. If your child is upset, don't force him to eat while he is crying. You may want him to finish his dinner or try something new, but if it leads to tears you are creating a choking hazard.

Don't allow sharing from plates. Your older child may want to help feed the baby or even let a younger sibling try something from her plate, but you need to teach them that this is not acceptable. Even adults might forget a potential choking hazard or to cut certain foods, so siblings shouldn't be expected to remember them either. Make it clear to kids as well as any adult who dines or supervises them that sharing from their plates is not allowed.

Take a cardiopulmonary resuscitation (CPR) class. It doesn't take very long and the lessons learned could save a life. You'll want to take a refresher course as your kids grow since techniques are different for older kids than for babies. The Red Cross offers classes. Go to *www.redcross.org* and check the links on the "Health and Safety Services" page. (See "Emergency Steps for a Choking Child," page 50.)

Keep carriers on the floor. Infant carriers can tip, so they should never be placed on a table, chair, counter, or any other high surface while occupied. Use them only on a level floor or ground. This means that if you feed your baby while she's in her carrier, you'll need to get down there with her. Be sure your little one is buckled into the carrier and it isn't tilted too far forward, which can block airways, or too far back, which can pose a choking risk.

Don't prop your carrier on a chair. Chairs and carriers were not designed to be used this way. There's no way to lock the carrier in place, and if someone bumps into your child the carrier can tip over.

Your child is ready for a high chair when he can hold his head up and his tummy is strong enough for him to sit up unaided. Otherwise, he might fall out.

Don't purchase a secondhand high chair. High chairs are being built sturdier and standards have become tougher over time. Many older chairs don't have a five-point harness or a post between the legs.

How to Buy a Safe High Chair

When shopping for a new high chair, look for these features to make sure the high chair is safe:

• A wide base, so the chair can't tip.
• A post that goes between the child's legs to prevent her from slipping between the seat and tray.
• A five-point harness system that consists of a waist belt, a belt that fits between your child's legs, and shoulder straps.

Five-point harness

Post between legs

Wheel locks

Wide base

Always use the high chair's harness, even if your child will be seated for only a few minutes. Children get fidgety, and your little bundle of energy is sure to try to escape from the chair at some point. The tray will not restrain her, so make sure the harness straps are snug so she can't get loose or become entangled, and check that the shoulder straps can't be pulled around her neck. If a restaurant gives you a chair with broken straps, ask for another chair.

Keep danger out of reach. Make sure your child can't reach the table, counter or potentially dangerous items from his high chair. You'd be surprised at what he can reach with one good stretch, especially from the sides of the chair or even from behind. As your child gets older, he may want to climb into the high chair himself. And since he is getting heavier too, you might be tempted to let him. Don't: The chair could tip over onto him. In fact, don't let any child play, climb, or lean on a high chair. Some kids like to use it as a jungle gym, but whether it's occupied or not, it's not a toy and should never be used for anything other than sitting and eating.

Hook-on chairs let you bring your baby right up to the table. Just be sure all dangerous items are out of her reach.

Make sure the chair is locked open. When using a foldable high chair, whether it is your own or one at a restaurant or some else's house, be sure the chair is locked into the fully opened position. Chairs can look fully opened and locked when they are not, so double check that the locking mechanism is fully engaged.

Take care with hook-on chairs. Be sure to follow the weight and height guidelines that you'll find in the owner's manual. Most have a weight range of 30 to 40 pounds. Before placing your baby in a hook-on chair, be sure the table is dry and the chair is secured to the table. Also make sure the chair is positioned so that your child can't dislodge it by pushing against another chair, bench, table leg or the table itself. Then belt your child into the chair. Be extra careful to keep such dangerous items as knives and forks out of his reach, not to mention anything breakable you don't want to get knocked onto the floor.

Not all tables are safe for hook-on chairs. Never use one with a table that has a glass top or a table that is supported by a single pedestal. Use these chairs only on sturdy, stable tables, and never with a tablecloth or placemat.

Secure that booster seat. First, attach it tightly to the chair using the set of straps provided for that purpose. Then strap your child to the booster using the waist belt and crotch strap. Make sure the chair is positioned so that your child can't push against chairs, benches or table supports to tip herself and the chair over.

The illustrated procedures below, based on information from the American Red Cross, are provided as a quick quide for what you should do if your child is choking. But it's no substitute for CPR training: The proper way to use this chart is in conjunction with CPR training. The Red Cross stresses that you should take first-aid and CPR training to learn the skills and build the confidence to act in an emergency.

First, if your child is coughing on something he swallowed, encourage him to continue coughing. If it gets to the point where your child can't cough, speak or breathe, that is when you need to step in. You should begin first aid for choking immediately if your child is wheezing, gurgling, turning blue, making a high-pitched noise, or clutching his throat. Have someone call 911 or the local emergency number.

The biggest difference between treating a choking infant and an adult is the position you should take and the force you should use. It is difficult to describe the force; there has to be some oomph behind it, but you don't want to go overboard with an infant. The Red Cross says that each back blow should be a separate and distinct attempt to dislodge the object. For more information on how to become trained in CPR, contact your local Red Cross chapter, or visit *www.redcross.org*.

Conscious Infant, Age 0-1

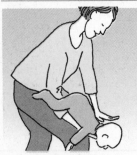

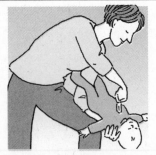

1. Give back blows.
Place your infant face-up on your forearm, then place the other arm on top so you are "sandwiching" the baby. While the baby is between your forearms, turn her facedown, with your forearm on your thigh. Give five firm back blows with the heel of your hand between your infant's shoulder blades.

2. Give chest thrusts.
If the object has not been forced out, cradle the infant between your forearms again and turn him over so he is facing up with his head lower than his chest. Place the pads of two or three fingers in the center of the baby's chest, between the nipples. Give five chest thrusts by compressing the breastbone ½ inch to 1 inch, and then letting the breastbone return to its normal position. Keep your fingers in place between chest thrusts. Alternate between sets of five back blows and five chest thrusts until the object is forced out, the infant begins to breathe on his own, or becomes unconscious.

If an Infant Becomes Unconscious

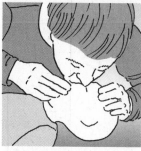

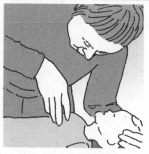

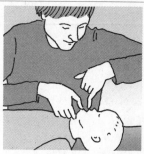

1. Give two breaths. If the infant becomes unconscious, cover his mouth and nose with your mouth and give two rescue breaths. Note: If you come upon an infant who is already unconscious from choking, start by giving 30 chest compressions as described in the next step. Give two breaths only after checking for an obstructing object as described in step 3.

2. Give chest compressions. If your breath does not go in, attempt to dislodge the object by giving 30 chest compressions. Compressions are given in the same way as chest thrusts, except you place the infant face-up on a flat surface, not on your knee.

3. Check for an obstructing object. After the 30 compressions, tip the infant's head back, open his mouth, hold his tongue down and look for the obstructing object. If you see an object try to sweep it out with your pinky. If you don't see anything or can't sweep it out, repeat steps 1-3, giving two breaths, then 30 chest compressions, then checking for an obstructing object, until the chest clearly rises with each rescue breath.

Conscious Child Age 1-12

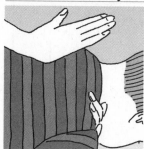

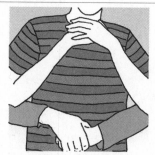

1. Give back blows. Position yourself slightly behind a child who is conscious but cannot cough, speak, or breathe. Provide support by placing one arm diagonally across the chest and lean the child forward. Give her five back blows

between the shoulder blades with your other hand. Each back blow should be a separate and distinct attempt to dislodge the object. If the back blows are not effective in forcing out the object, give five abdominal thrusts.

2. Give five abdominal thrusts. This is also known as the Heimlich maneuver. Stand or kneel behind the child and wrap your arms around his waist. Make a fist with one hand and place the thumb side against the middle of the child's abdomen, just above the navel and well below the lower tip of the breastbone. Grab your fist with your other hand and give quick, upward thrusts into the abdomen. Each abdominal thrust should be a separate attempt to dislodge the object. Continue back blows and abdominal thrusts until the object is dislodged and the child can breathe or cough forcefully, or becomes unconscious. *(Continued on page 52)*

If a Child Becomes Unconscious (Age 1-12)

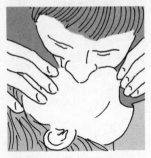 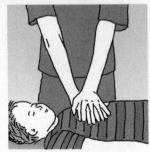 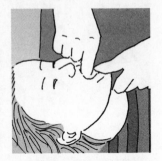

1. Give two breaths. Plug the child's nose and seal your mouth over his mouth. Pinch his nose while blowing air in and then release the nose. Note: If you come upon a child who already is unconscious, begin by giving 30 chest compressions as described in the next step. Give two breaths only after you have checked for an obstructing object as described in step 3.

2. Give 30 chest compressions. Place one or two hands in the center of the chest (on the lower half of the sternum). Compress the chest 1 ½ inches each time.

3. Check for an obstructing object. Open the child's mouth, hold his tongue down and look inside for an obstructing object. If you can see an object, sweep it out with your finger. If you can't see an object or are unable to sweep it out, give two breaths and begin again. Continue this process until the child begins to breathe on her own, you are too exhausted to continue, or a trained responder takes over for you.

CHAPTER 6

Living Room and Dining Room

Remember those pre-kid days when the living room was a place to kick back and relax, and the dining room was the venue for leisurely meals? Now your toddler is trying to dive off the couch or is hiding Cheerios under the sofa cushions. And you may think those are lovely silver candlesticks on the dining table, but Junior knows that they are actually laser swords. While the tips in this chapter won't restore pre-kid peace, they'll help you preserve your valuables while making sure the living room and dining room are places the entire family can safely enjoy.

Anchor any furniture that's on wheels. If furniture can move, your toddler will push against it and the next thing you know his legs will be out from under him. One good choice is to use those rubber coasters sold to protect floors from furniture feet. The coasters capture the wheels to prevent them from moving. Just be sure the pads are large enough not to be a choking hazard, and check periodically to be sure that they are securely fastened to the wheels and that no small pieces are loose.

Secure furniture that might tip. As your child begins to stand, she will try to use furniture to pull herself up. Anything that might potentially tip over should be secured to the walls or floor. This includes TV stands, bookcases, armoires, shelving units, and furniture stands. Be sure to secure these items before your little one is mobile. Some furniture comes with an anti-tip device, such as a strap or bracket, that you can secure to the furniture and fasten to the wall, but in many cases you'll have to purchase the device separately at a store or through a Web site that sells children's products. Be aware that the device must be secured into a wall stud—not just into drywall or plaster and lath. Otherwise, you can secure furniture to the floor using an L-bracket, also called an angle bracket. They can be found in any hardware store or home center.

Keep lamps out of your child's reach. Even a crawling infant can grab the cord and pull a lamp down on himself. One solution is to install a plastic cleat under the table and wrap one loop of the cord around it. You can find plastic cleats at hardware stores.

Make sure your TV can't tip. If it's in an enclosed unit, you should, of course, secure the unit to the wall using an anti-tip device. If your TV is on a separate stand, make sure the stand is no taller than 30 inches and designed specifically to hold a TV. Look for a UL (Underwriters Laboratories) sticker so you will know the stand meets current safety standards. And push the TV as far back on it as possible.

Whether enclosed unit or stand, the unit must be stable and strong enough to hold the weight of the TV. Your child will have a natural curiosity about the voices and picture coming through the TV. She might try to climb up the TV stand to turn on the TV, hit, touch or pull the TV, or grab a DVD player.

Never place your TV on top of a unit with drawers. This is a disaster waiting to happen. Your child can pull out the drawers and climb to the top, causing it to tip. Even if the unit is secured to the wall or floor, if he reaches the top, he might be able to slide the TV or DVD player onto the floor or worse, onto himself.

Keep wires out of reach. Your TV is probably hooked up to a DVR, cable or satellite, maybe a sound system or game console, or even a computer. The result can be a nest of wires. You'll want to keep those wires organized so you can tell which ones go where, but more important, so you can easily keep them well out of your youngster's reach to prevent her from trying to use them as a jump rope. Also, use a covered outlet strip to keep your child away from the plugs and outlets.

Keep little hands out of your electronics. Make sure your children can't get their hands inside any of those high-tech devices. Either keep your electronics in an enclosed cabinet or buy a guard that will prevent little hands from exploring them. Remember that your child sees you sticking videotapes and DVDs into those interesting gadgets, and he's bound to wonder what would happen if he inserted his hand or that spoon he smuggled from mealtime.

A covered power strip will keep curious toddlers away from plugs and outlets.

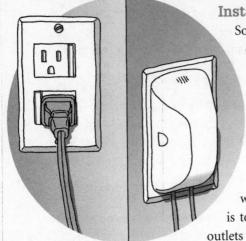

Install sliding outlet covers.

Some caps designed to keep fingers out of outlets are small enough to be a choking hazard. A better idea is to replace your outlet covers with ones that incorporate a panel that automatically slides closed when you remove a plug. To use the outlet, you have to use the plug to align the holes in the sliding panel with the outlet holes. Another option is to use a device that fully covers the outlets even when they are in use.

The outlet cover at left has panels that automatically slide over outlet holes that are not in use. Another option is a box that completely covers both outlets.

Keep furniture away from open windows. Your curious toddler or even an ambitious infant might use the couch as a ladder, possibly falling out of the window as he tries to get a better look at the outside world.

Install window guards. The outside world is an intriguing mystery to a small child. At some point he will figure out how to move that chair, sofa, or footstool over to the window. Properly installed window guards are another line of defense. Install the type that must be screwed into the window frame, and check them regularly to make sure the screws remain tight. Don't use pressure-mounted guards; a child can dislodge one by pushing or even just leaning on it. (See "Install window guards," page 3.)

Window stops are an alternative to window guards. (See "Window stops work, too," page 4.)

Use corner cushions. Do you have a coffee table or end tables with sharp corners? Use corner cushions to protect your crawler or toddler from scratches, cuts or worse. If your table is made of marble or another very hard material, use a table guard that wraps around the entire edge.

Make sure any glass tabletops in your home are made of tempered glass. Tempered glass is designed to shatter into small pieces if it breaks, instead of the more dangerous shards from regular glass. If you're buying a new table, the label might tell you whether the glass is tempered. If you are unsure about tables you already own, remove them.

Low tables made of very hard materials need wraparound table guards. For other tables, corner guards (inset) will do the job.

A tablecloth can be dangerous. Sure, a tablecloth or table runner looks great in a dining room, but to a toddler it might look just like another blanket. Sooner or later he's bound to pull it down, and if he does, whatever is on it might fall on top of him. One solution is to make sure there is nothing on the table or runner that could hurt your child if it falls. Otherwise, you can keep a tablecloth or runner folded shorter out of his reach, or just remove it from the table altogether.

Stools can tip. Do you have stools around your kitchen island or other eating area? Be aware that a fidgety child can easily tip a stool or even some chairs, by pushing his feet against the island or a table. Don't sit your child on a stool or lightweight chair until you are sure he understands the danger of tipping.

Are your dining chairs safe? Don't let your young child sit on a dining chair that has cutouts, is bentwood or has large slats in the back. Serious injury can result if your child's head or a limb becomes entrapped.

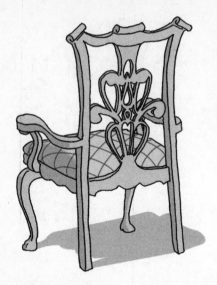

Secure your cabinets. If you have an armoire, breakfront or other cabinet in your dining room, fasten it to a wall using an anti-tip device or safety strap so when your little one decides she wants to have an unauthorized tea party with your china, she can't tip the cabinet. Also, consider adding a childproof lock to the cabinet doors.

Install gates before your child is mobile. Once he starts crawling you'll have your hands full trying to stop him from exploring every corner of your home.

Don't allow a small child to sit in any chair with spaces large enough to fit an arm, a leg or his head.

Some gates are pressure mounted, that is, they have parts that press against a wall, stairway rail or doorframe to keep it in place. Others are attached to a wall or doorframe with hardware. Some models can be installed either way. Pressure-mounted gates are handy because you can move them as needed and you don't have to drill any holes in your walls. But they are not as secure as hardware-mounted gates. Use pressure-mounted gates only in areas where falling isn't a major concern, such as between two rooms with same-level flooring or the bottom of stairs. Whichever type of gate you use, be certain it is secure. Even hardware-mounted gates should be checked to make sure the mounting screws have not come loose.

Use only hardware-mounted gates at the top of stairs. This type of gate provides the most secure barrier because you install it with brackets that are solidly screwed into a doorframe or into wood studs in the wall. If there is baseboard or other molding where you plan to install a gate, you might need a gate-mounting kit to compensate for the molding's thickness and provide you with a flat mounting surface.

Are You Living with Poisonous Plants?

Those plants or cut flowers in your living room may be poisonous, and it only takes a moment for your child to grab a leaf or flower or find one that has fallen and put it in her mouth. Here is the National Capital Poison Center's list of poisonous plants that could be in your home. Many of the plants grow outdoors, but they are included here so you'll know not to cut their blossoms for indoor display and you can be aware of them when your kids are playing outdoors. You can see photos of some of these plants at *www.poison.org*.

If you have a plant that isn't on this list, that doesn't mean it isn't poisonous. To be sure, you can call your local poison center at 800-222-1222. If you find you have poisonous plants in your home, get rid of them.

- Azalea
- Rhododendron
- Caladium
- Castor bean
- Daffodil (Narcissus)
- Deadly nightshade (Belladonna)
- Dumb cane
- Elephant Ear
- Foxglove
- Fruit pits and seeds
- Holly
- Iris
- Jerusalem cherry
- Jimson weed
- Lantana
- Lily-of-the-valley
- May apple
- Mistletoe
- Morning glory
- Mountain laurel
- Nightshade
- Oleander
- Peace lily
- Philodendron
- Pokeweed
- Pothos
- Yew (Taxus)

Keep all houseplants and flower arrangements out of your child's reach. Regularly pinch off dead or loose leaves and discard wilted flowers. If leaves, berries, or petals fall, discard them immediately.

If the gate will be at the top of the stairs, look for one that swings in only one direction and install it so that it opens away from the stairwell.

Install gates safely. Purchase a tall enough gate designed for children rather than pets. Some gates have an expanding pressure bar that a child could use to climb over, so be sure to install them with the bar outside the room your child will be in. And if you need to step on a pedal or button to open your gate, be aware that your child will be watching and trying to learn this behavior. Sooner or later, he will figure it out.

Don't use old accordion-style child gates. They have V-shaped openings along the top and diamond-shaped openings below that are large enough to entrap a child's head, creating a strangulation hazard. Likewise, don't use circular wooden enclosures that expand accordion style because they present a similar hazard.

Use swings safely. If you have a baby swing in your living room, check that it is fully open and locked before each use and that it isn't near furniture, curtains, wires, or lamps that she can grab. Many swings have a reclined position and an infant headrest to help keep your baby's head properly positioned. Don't remove this headrest or use the swing in the upright position until you are sure your baby can hold her head up on her own. If her head falls forward, her airway can become obstructed.

Buckle in your child before using a baby swing. Don't rely on a tray or other support devices to keep your child in the swing. As she gets older she may try to make a break for it, so make sure your swing has a five-point harness to keep her safely in place.

Make sure the swing is placed on a flat, stable surface. Never place it on an elevated surface. Set the swing for a slow speed at first; as your baby gets older and more used to the swing, you can adjust the speed. Limit swing time to 30 minutes and make sure the speed setting isn't too fast.

Never move the swing with your child in it. If you want to change location, remove your child first. A swing is not an infant carrier and was not designed to carry your child.

Know when your child has outgrown the swing. Most

No Gate Hopping Allowed!

Get into the habit of opening and closing your gate rather than climbing over it. You'll be safer—it's easier to stumble than you think—and you won't be giving your kids the idea that gates can be climbed over.

babies love swings, and using one gives you a chance to relax and catch your breath. Be aware, though, that baby swings have weight and height limits. Check your owner's manual; most limit weight to 25 or 30 pounds. And if your child tries to escape from the swing or is too active in it, stop using it. This goes for any baby product with safety restraints. If your child wants to get out, sooner or later he will find a way.

Walkers can increase your baby's exposure to hazards. The American Academy of Pediatrics recommends that if you have a walker you should dispose of it. Walkers can give a child access you don't want him to have to areas of the home, such as the kitchen stove or the fireplace. Instead of a walker, you may want to try a stationary activity center. This will allow your child to play while giving you some hands-free time without the need to chase your speed racer around the house. However, don't leave your baby in a stationary activity center for more than 30 minutes because it's not good for her growing body.

If you insist on using a walker, closely supervise your baby while she is in it. Walkers are required to have some kind of mechanism to keep them from going down a staircase. There are two common devices intended to do this. One is a bumper that makes the walker too wide to fit through a 36-inch doorway—the idea is to prevent your child from zooming out of a room toward a staircase. If you'll use the walker in rooms with doorways that are wider than 36-inches, look for a walker with the second common device: a friction strip that is sup-posed to stop the walker at the edge of a stairway. However, CONSUMER

REPORTS' testing has found that these strips don't always work, so be sure to keep your child away from stairs while she is in a walker. Also be aware that walkers have weight restrictions, which you will find in the owner's manual.

Walkers require constant vigilance. Even if you live in a single-story house or have effectively blocked walker access to your stairs, you'll still need to keep an eagle eye on your child to keep her from scooting into trouble. There's the fireplace, or the pool, or a lamp waiting to be pulled off an end table. There's a letter opener on the desk, a knife on the table, a hairdryer in the bathroom or myriad other dangerous things waiting to be grabbed.

Wait until your baby is ready. Don't use your stationary activity center or walker until your baby can hold his head up on his own and can sit up unassisted. Stop using it when he reaches the weight or height limit (usually 30 inches or 30 pounds; check the owner's manual), or when he begins to walk, whichever comes first.

Keep your stationary activity center away from hazards in a room, such as furniture, curtains, lamps, cords, hot surfaces or sources of water. Keep a watchful eye on your child as she plays, and check the activity center's toys for wear.

An activity center might not always be stationary. Even though stationary activity centers are supposed to stay in one place, your baby may be able to move it a bit as he gets bigger and more active. Keep this in mind and keep him out of the path of potential dangers.

Keep your activity center on the ground. Just like all juvenile products, it should be on a flat, level surface. Don't carry the activity center with your child in it, and always make sure there aren't any broken parts or missing pieces. Your activity center may also have stabilizers to prevent it from bouncing. They should be sturdy so they don't release unexpectedly.

Limit bouncer time. While you are sitting in your living room, you might decide to put your infant in a bouncer seat to give him some play-time and yourself some hands-free time. Bouncer seats usually consist of a lightweight flexible frame covered with cloth that conforms to your baby's body. Just as a walker, swing and stationary activity center shouldn't be used as a baby-sitter, neither should your bouncer seat. It's best to limit this activity to 30 minutes as well.

Make sure your baby is ready to bounce. When using a bouncer, check whether it has adequate head support. This head support should be removable, so you can take it off when your child can hold her head up on her own.

All bouncer seats have weight limits. Most have a limit of approximately 25 pounds, some less, some more. You should stop using the seat if your child can lean forward or stand up unassisted because she might tip the seat forward. Check the restrictions in your owner's manual.

Check your bouncer for wear and tear before each use. Make sure there are no holes in the fabric and that the toys on the toy bar aren't loose.

Use your bouncer only on a level floor or ground. Never place it on a chair, table, bed or any elevated surface because it could fall off the edge. Or if the surface is not level or if it is soft like a bed, the bouncer could tip over. Although a bed is a soft surface to tip onto, your child could suffocate in the bedding.

Make sure the toy bar is secured. If your bouncer has a toy bar that locks, make sure it is firmly in place so your baby can't release it. Some

✴ Living Room and Dining Room

63

toy bars are heavy and can hurt your infant if she kicks it off. Never carry your baby in the bouncer because the framework may not support her weight. And remember that the toy bar is not a handle.

Older products can be risky. Standards for children's products have become more stringent over time. For example, some older products don't have up-to-date restraint systems. So it's best to purchase new products. If you are using a product for a second child, check to see if it has been recalled or if the newer version has tougher, sturdier parts and restraints.

CHAPTER 7

The Playroom

When you have kids, it might feel like every room in your house has turned into a playroom. Toys seem to magically multiply and take over your home. The best way to reclaim your house is to make one room or small area into the playroom or play area. Even more important than helping you stay organized, you'll be creating a special environment that's safe and kid-friendly.

Organize the room. When you're having a tough day, just getting the toys put away seems like a major accomplishment. Organization is the key to making it easier. As a first step in organizing the playroom, get on your hands and knees and try to see the room from your child's perspective. This will help you determine how best to store his toys as well as identify the potential dangers in the playroom. Organize the room so your child can easily reach his toys, thus eliminating the temptation to climb to get something he wants and allowing him to safely explore his space. Lots of handy storage makes it easy to put toys away where no one can trip over them.

Beware of hinged lids. Toy chests or storage bins with hinged lids can fall on your child's head or neck, trapping her or causing serious injury. And children have been known to crawl into these chests and suffocate while trapped inside.

If you have a toy chest, or any chest, with a freely falling hinged lid, the safest thing you can do is remove the lid entirely. Or you can add a lid support; heavy lids may require two.

If the lid on your toy chest can slam shut, install one or two lid supports to prevent injury to your child.

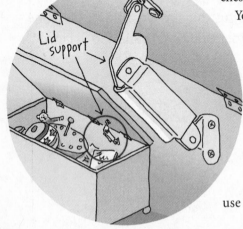

Lid support →

A lid support will keep the lid of the toy chest open in any position you choose. You can purchase a chest with a lid support or one that has hinges that support the lid, or you can install a lid support or two yourself. Check them frequently to ensure they are still in good working order and that they do indeed work in any position. Remember to check, tighten, and adjust as necessary.

For easy storage alternatives, use baskets or open bins.

Don't Use These Recalled Chests

In 1996, 12 million cedar chests made by Lane and Virginia Maid were recalled after six children became trapped inside and suffocated because the lids automatically latched when closed. The chests were made between 1912 and 1987, and many have been handed down as heirlooms, and they can still be found at yard sales or in secondhand stores.

Even since this recall there have been two near fatalities and one fatal accident. The Consumer Product Safety Commission (CPSC) and Lane are still working to recall these chests. As a remedy, Lane is providing new locks for the old chests that will prevent entrapment, and the company will provide assistance to anyone who needs help installing the new lock. To find out if you have a Lane chest that has been recalled and to request a lock replacement, check the Lane Web site at *www.lanefurniture.com* and click on "customer care."

Make toys accessible. When storing toys, use baskets, buckets, or other containers that allow your child to easily reach inside to pull out what she needs. Be sure the toys in these containers are age-appropriate for all of your children. A 2-year-old should not share toys that are for a 6-year-old because of the danger to the younger child from small toy parts that could pose a choking hazard.

Don't tempt fate by placing your young child's toys and games on high shelves or ledges in the playroom. It's more than likely that he will figure out how to climb up to get them, with potentially deadly results. If he is allowed to have the toys, store them within his reach. If he shouldn't have them, keep them out of sight.

Always check the age recommendation on the packaging of a toy before you allow it in your playroom. The age grading relates to safety as well as play value.

Toys labeled for children 3 and older may have small parts and pieces that can be a choking hazard for children younger than that. If you have a child younger than 3, don't buy a toy with a warning that it is not for a young child. Never give a child under the age of 3 a toy that is recommended for an older child; some toys may need to stay in the closet until your child reaches the appropriate age. Even if your child is 3 years old, you may want to hold off giving her toys that will fit in her mouth.

When in doubt, ask. If you're not sure about the age appropriateness of a toy, check with the manufacturer. In addition, if a small piece that can be ingested has broken off one of your toys labeled for a child who is less than 3 years old, call the manufacturer and the U.S. Consumer Product Safety Commission (CPSC) at 800-638-2772 to report the incident. Even if your child has not swallowed the detached part, reporting the toy may help prevent a future disaster.

Electric toys must be age-appropriate. Electric toys are regulated by the CPSC for the safe and durable enclosure of electrical devices as well as maximum surface temperature. Even though these regulations are in place, check the package for the minimum age. You should buy an electric toy only for a child who is mature enough to use it safely and only with your supervision.

Don't service toys with kids around. Wait until naptime, or bedtime, or until someone else is supervising your kids so they won't be around screwdrivers, batteries, screws, and other small components.

Make Organizing Fun

You can turn the job of organizing a playroom into a fun project for you and your child. It's simple: Buy some sturdy plastic containers with lids that snap closed. Working together, fill the containers with different items, such as books in one, toy cars in another, and toy animals in another. Next, look in magazines for photos of the items in your containers and cut them out. Using glue labeled "nontoxic," "washable," or "for school use," attach the photos onto the corresponding containers. Glue is recommended only for kids over 5, so make sure you're supervising if your child is younger than that.

Move toys up. Keep toys that aren't age-appropriate—such as puzzles or board games with small pieces—on higher shelves or in an area, such as a closet, your toddler can't reach. It is important to keep these toys out of sight as well so your toddler won't be tempted to try to reach them. Again, teach your older child that these toys are only for her, and she can play with them during her little brother's naptime or when another adult is watching her younger sib.

Look for little pieces. Check toys for small or detachable pieces. Do they have small buttons or eyes that can be removed by a curious 2-year-old? Do they have small plastic pieces that can easily be ingested? When in doubt, save the toy for when your child is older. Three-year-olds pull, prod and twist toys. Look for ones that are well made with tightly secured eyes, noses and other parts. Avoid toys that have sharp edges and points.

Avoid items that can be broken into smaller pieces, such as chalk or crayons, or that have detachable components, such as caps from markers and pens. You will be amazed at what your child will put in his mouth. Small pieces of larger toys are just as dangerous as small toys themselves.

Watch for small parts. The battle against toys with small pieces is larger than you may realize. Your older child might have jewelry, marbles, small puzzle pieces, balls, dress-up dolls with small shoes, or action figures with small components. None of this is appropriate for his sisters and brothers under 3 years old. Constantly monitor the older sibling's toys, and remind your little one never to put any of these items in her mouth.

Expect the unexpected. Check small toy trucks and cars for wheels or components that may dislodge. Be sure the rubber tips on the ends of drumsticks are intact. Make sure buttons on stuffed animals and small pieces on electronic toys haven't become displaced. Toys have been recalled for all of those reasons and many more.

Small Magnets Can Cause Serious Injury

Small, powerful magnets can cause serious health problems and even death if swallowed or inhaled. Two or more swallowed magnets (or one magnet and a small metal object, such as a steel ball or a metal charm) can attract one another through intestinal walls. The magnets will not pass through the body but instead will become trapped. They can twist or pinch the intestine, causing holes, blockage and infection in the intestine or blood poisoning, all of which can be fatal. Surgery is required to remove trapped magnets from the intestines.

Unfortunately, the non-specific abdominal symptoms are often misdiagnosed. They include abdominal pains, nausea, vomiting, and diarrhea.

If your child shows any of those symptoms, or if you suspect that he has ingested magnets, seek immediate medical attention. Tell the doctor that you suspect magnets may be the cause and ask for an X-ray.

To avoid this hazard, remove small magnets and any toys that contain them from your child's playroom, no matter what your child's age. Small magnets have been known to fall out of toys and other objects. For this reason, allow no magnets—separate or contained within toys—unless the magnets themselves are too large to fit through a toilet paper tube.

If you find loose, small magnets around the house, track down the source. Immediately take the product and any of its other magnetic components away from your child and contact the manufacturer and the Consumer Product Safety Commission at 800-638-2772 or go to *www.cpsc.gov.*

Check the play area. Make sure your child hasn't appropriated small objects, such as coins from the sofa, or a plastic bag.

Beware of sharp objects. Remove anything with a sharp point, such as a colored pencil. Sharp edges are prohibited on toys for any child under age 8, so discard any that have them. Wooden toys that have become sharp or splintered can be sanded.

No-name products may be no bargain. If a juvenile product or toy doesn't have a manufacturer's name and a model number, it will be difficult or impossible to check if the product has been recalled. This can be a problem with items purchased at dollar stores, thrift stores, yard sales, or vending machines.

Discard cheap jewelry. The CPSC has recalled millions of pieces of jewelry for lead-poisoning hazards. It's difficult to distinguish lead-laden jewelry from nonlead pieces, so discard any cheap jewelry you may have now.

Do your own choking-hazard test. If your child is less than 3 years old, or if you notice he is still putting toys in his mouth, make sure any toys you give him are too big to fit through a toilet-paper tube. Manufacturers do a similar test with a smaller tube. The more-stringent toilet-paper tube test will further ensure that you don't give your children toys that are a choking hazard. (See "Emergency Steps for a Choking Child," page 50.)

Beware of balls. Choking caused by small balls has long been a leading cause of death attributed to toys. Balls less than 1¼ inches in diameter can pose a choking hazard to young children. If a ball can fit through a toilet-paper tube, you don't want it in the play-room if your child is less than 3 years old or still putting things in his mouth.

Get rid of balloons. Of all children's products, balloons are the leading cause of suffocation death, according to the CPSC. They have been associated with more than 110 deaths since 1973. If a child takes a breath while trying to blow up a balloon, the bal-loon can be drawn back into her mouth and may seal off her airway, creating a tighter, more lethal seal, with each attempt to breathe. Children can suffocate even while chew-ing or sucking on a balloon. Popped balloons are hazardous

To prevent choking in children under 3 years old, don't give them any toy that can't fit through a toilet-paper tube.

Watch Out for Lead

Lead has been found in toys and in a wide array of products that your children may come in contact with.

To learn how you can minimize your children's exposure, see Keeping the Lead Out, page 187.

too; a small piece can cause the same type of airway obstruction as an entire balloon.

Use doll apparatus for dolls, not children. Play cribs, bassinets, and strollers are fun, but don't let your child try to sit in any of them or try to put a younger sibling in one. They are not designed to hold a child's weight. A child could get hurt if the stroller, crib, or bassinet collapses while she is inside, or she could become trapped in an opening that is meant to hold a doll, not secure a child.

Small play food can be hazardous. If you have a play kitchen, be sure the plastic food is age-appropriate. Play food is designed for children over age 3. It looks very realistic, and toddlers may try to eat some. Be sure you are giving your younger child play food that is large and can't be accidentally swallowed. If your older child sticks everything in his mouth, the food is enticing, or you worry about accidental ingestion, you may want to stick to the large play food for your older child as well.

Keep play in the play kitchen. Be sure your child knows that the knives and forks in her play kitchen and the plastic pots, pans, and kettles on her play stove are pretend. Play kitchens are not recommended for children under 3. Real utensils should always be off-limits, whether you're in your kitchen or dining in a restaurant. You don't want her to reach for your real pots and pans one day.

Be cautious with play clothes. Kids begin enjoying dress-up outfits as early as 1 year old. Until they are 3, however, anything they wear should be smooth and large enough so it can't be swallowed. Watch out for buttons, beads, tassels, pom-poms, bows, or any other small pieces that could come loose and pose a choking hazard. Don't allow necklaces until age 4.

Play clothes and accessories belong inside. Costume jewelry and dress-up outfits are meant for the playroom, not for the playground. When your youngster does start wearing costume jewelry and dress-up outfits, be sure she wears them in the house (though not in the crib or play yard) and not on the playground, where they can get tangled or caught on slides, swings, and jungle gyms, or on the school bus.

Avoid cords and strings. Pull toys are fun and so are toy telephones, but both usually have a string or cord attached. Avoid toys with cords or strings, or be sure the cord or string is very short so it can't become wrapped around your child's neck. Take extra precautions and cut off the straps or strings if necessary. Toy guitars with a strap or a toy stethoscope can be dangerous because the strap goes around the neck, so such a toy should not be given to young children.

Ban flying objects. Use projectiles with caution; this type of toy can cause injury. Arrows or darts should have soft cork tips, rubber suction cups or other protective devices attached. Even so, these should be used only with supervision and never by children younger than 8.

Keep caps out of pockets. Don't let your kids put ring caps, paper roll caps or strip caps for toy guns in their pockets. Friction can ignite the caps and cause burns. Keep caps away from children under 8.

Toy tools need to be the right size. Toy tools, such as rakes and shovels, should be lightweight and fit your child's hand. A toy that is too large or too tall can be dangerous for a small child.

Purchase washable toys. If your little one loves to put things in her mouth, buy washable toys that are meant to withstand mouthing and be sure to keep them clean.

Keep crafts safe. Kids love arts and crafts as they get older. Work with your child and be sure the materials you choose are age-appropriate. When purchasing arts and crafts materials, stay away from permanent paints and markers. Look for water-based washable paints and glues. For a child under 3 years old or one who still puts things in his mouth, purchase age-appropriate material that can't be swallowed—no beads, small foam pieces or small pom-pom balls.

Remember the scissors rules. Make sure your scissors are age-appropriate, and don't give any type of scissors to a child under age 3. The scissors should be blunt. The packaging will often say "safety scissors" and will provide age guidelines. Remember that even child-friendly scissors should be used only with adult supervision. Be sure your child knows how to use them safely and properly. Teach him to keep them pointed downward with his hand closed around them when he walks, and never to run with them.

Remove play-yard hazards. Don't add pillows or an additional mattress to your play yard, also known as a playpen, or travel bed. The additional mattress on top can very easily shift, causing a space that can trap your child; pillows pose a suffocation hazard. Use only the play-yard mattress that comes with the equipment. It should be no more than 1 inch thick, and it must fit snugly to prevent your child from becoming trapped between the mattress and the mesh side. If you want to use a sheet on the mattress, use one that is made for that play-yard mattress.

Pay attention to bedding. The only bedding that should go in the play yard is the mattress. Never use adult sheets, blankets or quilts, or toys with strings or cords. Put your child to sleep on her back in the play yard, just as you would in a crib. Think of the play yard as a big bed that she plays in; the safety rules for a bed don't change just because the bed is on the floor and the sides of the bed are made of mesh.

Make sure your play yard is properly set up and in good shape before placing your child in it.

Look for play-yard problems.

Frequently check your play yard for possible tears, holes, or threads in the mesh. The mesh weave should be small, with individual holes of no more than ¼ inch in diameter. Discard the play yard if you find tears or large holes, which are an entrapment hazard. Make sure the mesh is attached securely to the rails.

Look over the play yard very carefully with an eye for hazards—basically anything that could trap a child, be it a hanging strap or a gap between the sides and the floorboard. Check your play yard for any other potential hazards, such as loose fabric in the bassinet that could entrap an infant, any straps that hang down from an attached changing table, or protruding rivets that could catch clothing. If your play yard was recalled, bring it back to the store for a refund or replacement.

Check play-yard locks. Current safety standards require that play-yard top rails lock automatically into place when the play yard is set up. If you have to rotate the rails into a locked position, your play yard may have been recalled. If you bought your play yard at a yard sale or it was a hand-me-down, you might have a play yard with this problem. If you have any doubt, check the Consumer Product Safety Commission Web

The Playroom

site at *www.cpsc.gov* and the manufacturer's Web site for recalls. If you don't see your play yard on the list, you can play it extra safe by calling the manufacturer and giving them your make and model number to be sure your play yard has not been recalled.

Avoid older play yards. Don't purchase a second-hand play yard and don't use other people's play yards when you go on trips or play dates unless you know that specific model hasn't been recalled. Also check it for any hazards yourself. If you plan to use a play yard provided by a hotel, inquire about the model before your trip. Safety standards have improved and play yards have become safer over the years, which means that many older models are no longer considered safe.

Keep the sides up. Never leave your child in his play yard with one of the sides in the down position. He could get trapped between the rails or escape the play yard. Also, remove attachments, such as bassinets and changing tables, before placing the child in the play yard.

Childproof your playroom. Be sure all bookcases, TV stands, and wall units are properly fastened to the wall (see "Use furniture restraints," page 9) and plug up all electrical outlets with safety covers that replace the original outlet cover (see "Install sliding outlet covers," page 56). Cover corners and sharp edges with corner guards or cushioning (see "Use corner cushions," page 56).

Check Out This Checklist for Hotel Play Yards and Cribs

The CPSC has created two handy one-page checklists to help you make sure that any hotel-supplied crib or play yard you use is safe.

Print out both checklists before you hit the road. You'll find them at *www.cpsc.gov/cpscpub/pubs/5136.pdf.*

CHAPTER 8

The Backyard

As soon as your kids step out the back door, they enter a whole new world of potential hazards: from poisonous plants to fish ponds, to toxic gardening supplies and more, not to mention the challenge of keeping them safe as they climb and swing on the backyard play set. Here are some simple precautions you'll need to make sure the backyard is a safe place to play.

Always supervise. No matter how safe you think your young ones are on your own property, an accident can occur in a matter of seconds. You should keep a watchful eye on them at all times during play, and if you need to run into the house, they should come with you. Unsupervised play is unsafe.

Even a bucket can be dangerous. Pay attention to everyday outdoor items that can quickly turn into safety hazards. A five-gallon bucket used to clean outdoor furniture or for yard work may seem harmless, but it can quickly fill with rainwater and pose a drowning danger to an infant or toddler. The same is true of a plastic trash can or anything else that can hold water. Empty any vessel after each use—even an inch or two of water can be dangerous—and either turn it over or bring it inside the house when you're done with it.

Remove dead tree branches. While a spot under a shady tree is nice for playing, picnicking, reading, or relaxing, the branches that lend cover may be more dangerous than they look. A falling tree branch can cause serious injuries or even death to both children and adults. Have all dead branches taken down and all dead trees removed from your property. If the tree is not on your property, talk to your neighbors about the hazard. If you are renting, talk to your landlord. They may thank you for bringing it to their attention. No one wants to see a child or anyone else get hurt this way. If you can't remove dead trees or branches, don't allow your children to play under them or anywhere near them.

Prune lower limbs. Be sure to cut all tree limbs up to 7 feet off the ground. Even though you bought a nice new swing set for your child, he will probably still want to use the tree as a jungle gym. He can suffer a dangerous fall from one or get stuck while climbing.

Cover window wells. You don't want your child to fall into a window well while trying to retrieve a ball. A fall into a window well could lead to a broken limb or even a broken neck. Cover wells with a sturdy plastic cover made for that purpose. They can be made to fit your specific window well, and should withstand the weight of a child. Still, teach your children not to stand on or play on these covers.

Don't let your child wear clothes with drawstrings. These can lead to choking or strangulation on outdoor play equipment. Although the CPSC has created a voluntary standard for clothing manufacturers that prohibits drawstrings, you still may come across them. If you find an item with a drawstring, remove it and call the CPSC Consumer Hotline at 800-638-2772, or go to *www.cpsc.gov* to report the article of clothing.

Clear plastic covers made to fit your window wells let light into the basement while eliminating the possibility that children will fall in.

Scarves, jewelry, and purse straps are dangerous. They can get stuck or tangled in play equipment. While your daughter may want to get all decked out for a play date in the yard, don't let her play on outdoor equipment with jewelry, purses, or scarves.

Beware of burns from metal play equipment. Check slides and other metal play equipment. The sun can make these surfaces hot enough to cause second- or third-degree burns in a matter of seconds.

Be careful of entrapment hazards. Be sure that any platforms or ramps have guardrails. The spacing in guardrails or between ladder rungs should be either too big or too small to entrap a child. The spacing should measure less than 3½ inches or more than 9 inches.

Set Up That Play Set Correctly

Properly installed play sets are a good, safe way for kids to have fun and get exercise while you supervise them from the comfort of your own yard. Here are some tips for safe installation of play sets:

• Do not install your play set over grass. Injury from a fall onto grass can be just as bad as a fall onto concrete. Place your play set over loose fill with dirt beneath. Do not install loose fill over concrete or asphalt. The Consumer Product Safety Commission recommends using wood mulch or chips, engineered wood fiber (EFW), or mulch of shredded recycled rubber for equipment up to 8 feet high, or sand or pea gravel for equipment up to 5 feet high.

• Make the fill at least 12 inches deep. You'll need to replace fill as it compacts, washes away or deteriorates. Don't let it get less than 9 inches deep. Be aware that wood chips deteriorate quicker than nonwood fills and that mulch deteriorates even quicker than chips. Mark the correct level on the play equipment support posts so you can see when the fill drops below.

• To order your loose fill, you need to know the area of the use zone—under and around a play set where children might fall. The total use zone depends on the type of play equipment. In general, the surface should extend at least 6 feet in all directions from the edge of the stationary equipment.

• For a slide with a platform up to 4 feet high, play-area surfacing needs to cover 6 feet at the sides and exit of the slide. For slides with a platform higher than 4 feet, you need 6 feet at the sides and 8 feet at the front.

• The use zone for swings is twice the height of the swing hanger (the top bar of the swing seat) in front and in back of the swing seats. For example, if the hanger height is 8 feet, the use zone must be 16 feet in front and 16 feet in back of the hanger. Surfacing should also extend 6 feet to each side of the swing.

• Frequently check your play set for missing, loose, or rusting hardware, chains, and S-hooks. The CPSC recommends that you check all bolts and screws twice a month and tighten them as needed.

• If you need to replace hardware on your set, purchase it from the manufacturer of your swing set. Do not replace the hardware with nuts or bolts purchased from the local hardware store, because they are not made to withstand the same stresses, weight, and wear-and-tear as hardware made specifically for a play set.

• If the play set has a platform, make sure the platform has a protective barrier or guardrail to prevent curious kids from falling—or more adventurous children from leaping off it.

• The seats on your swings should be made of rubber, not metal or wood.

Children have been known to dash in front of a moving swing, and a heavy metal or wood swing seat could cause a serious head injury.

• Play equipment for children between the ages of 6 months and 23 months should be no higher than 32 inches and should have a use zone of 4 feet in all directions. Only you can judge if your child is even ready for this equipment, and you or a caretaker must be within arm's reach at all times.

• If you have any questions regarding the safety of your play set or proper installation, visit the Web site for the National Program for Playground Safety, at *www.playgroundsafety.org* or call 800-554-PLAY(7529).

• For more detailed information about planning, constructing, and maintaining a home playground, download the U.S. Consumer Product Safety Commission's Outdoor Home Playground Safety Handbook. Find it at *www.cpsc.gov/CPSC PUB/PUBS/324.pdf*.

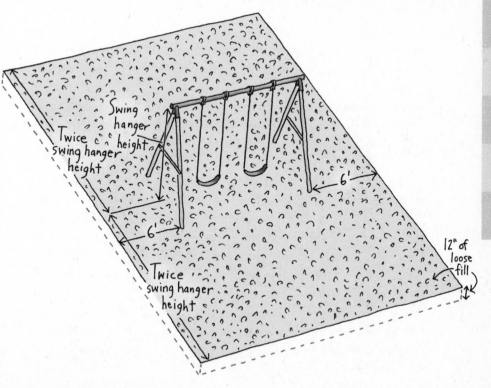

Swing hanger height

Twice Swing hanger height

Twice swing hanger height

6'

6'

12" of loose fill

Know Trampoline Dangers and Guidelines

• Many pediatricians consider trampolines too dangerous to use. CONSUMER REPORTS agrees. The CPSC estimates that in 2006, there were 109,522 injuries associated with trampolines that required emergency room visits, including 69,000 children between the ages of 2 and 11. If you insist on owning a trampoline, you should follow these important guidelines:
• Supervise children at all times.
• Don't allow children under age 6 to use the trampoline.
• Enclose the trampoline so that children don't accidentally bounce off.

• Cover all exposed bars, springs, and hooks with shock-absorbing padding.
• Allow only one child at a time to jump on the trampoline.
• Don't allow somersaults; landing on the head or neck can result in serious injury, even paralysis.
• Make sure the trampoline is placed far away from trees, structures, and play areas.
• Don't use a ladder; young children can use it to climb on the trampoline at unsupervised times.

Stick with the standard equipment. Don't attach anything other than the recommended playground equipment to your play set. Don't allow your child to attach jump ropes or any other kind of rope, pet leashes, or clotheslines to your play equipment. While using play equipment, kids shouldn't have purses, necklaces, or anything else with long strings or ties that could cause strangulation.

Take precautions with play sets made of treated wood. If you have a wooden play set that was purchased before the end of 2003 and the it is not made of redwood or cedar, the wood was most likely pressure-treated with chromated copper arsenate (CCA) to prevent rotting. CCA contains arsenic, which can leech from the wood, so the first precautions to take are to prohibit eating while using the play set and make sure children wash their hands after using it.

You can reduce CCA leeching by applying water-based or oil-based outdoor stain to the wood once a year. Don't use paint, which requires sanding that will produce CCA-leaden dust. Unlike paint, stain soaks in and won't peel off.

Insist on shoes. It is difficult to be certain that your backyard is free of hidden hazards, such as broken glass, cans, metal, nails, or wood slivers from a deck, so make sure your kids keep their shoes on outdoors. Shoes also protect them from hot surfaces that could burn feet, and from insects in grass. (Bees really like clover.) Children love to play barefoot and they probably won't notice these hazards as they toss a ball, chase a friend, or play hide-and-go-seek.

Cover the sandbox when not in use. Your sandbox can become a repository for all sorts of hidden hazards. You can't see what your child or another child has dropped into the sandbox. Periodically rake or sift the sand just to make sure there aren't any unexpected surprises in there. Also remember that a sandbox is attractive for animals to use when we aren't looking. Buy or make a cover to keep the sand in and everything else out.

Keep kids away from fish ponds. A fish pond or a fountain can be intriguing to a curious toddler. If water pools at the bottom of the fountain, you need to keep children away from it and teach them not to lean in for a closer look. A larger pond should be treated as a pool: Surround it with fencing at least 4 feet high, and make sure there's a self-closing, self-latching gate.

Check your backyard for poisonous plants. Many popular backyard trees, shrubs and plants have leaves and/or flowers that are poisonous. (See "Are You Living with Poisonous Plants," page 59.) Remove these plants from areas where children play.

Don't Donate Your Play Set for Public Use

Your home play set was made to meet a different standard than one designed to be used more often by a larger group of children. Despite your good intentions, it can't be reused by schools, or daycare facilities. Their play sets must meet a recognized industry standard.

Store dangerous gardening items inside. The best place to store your garden tools, plant food, pesticides, and paints is in locked cabinets in your garage, out of your children's reach. If you don't have garage space, or if you have items that can be ruined by temperature extremes (latex paint, for example, shouldn't be allowed to freeze), store in locked cabinets in the house, out of your children's reach. Never store dangerous items so they are accessible on a shelf or in containers in the backyard, no matter how secure you think those containers might be.

Use nontoxic gardening supplies. The American Academy of Pediatrics recommends using nontoxic fertilizers, insecticides, and gardening supplies. Labels will give you an idea of how hazardous a product can be. Products labeled "danger" are the most hazardous, followed by "warning," and then "caution." Try to avoid products bearing these labels.

Secure your workshop. If your garage doubles as a workshop, keep all tools out of your child's reach and make the garage off-limits unless you are there with your child. Be sure to discard toxic and flammable materials that you no longer need. Do not store flammable liquids, such as paints, paint thinners and cleaners, near any heat sources. Keep all such materials locked up and in their original containers, so that if a child does ingest something you'll know what it is.

Don't use power tools around kids. Do not mow the lawn, trim the hedges, edge the walk, or use any other gas- or electric-powered tools when children are in the yard. These tools are simply too dangerous. Don't let kids ride on a lawn mower or play on it when it is stored.

Practice caution around the barbecue. Adults should remain vigilant to keep kids away from the barbecue when it is in use. Always lock up propane tanks, lighter fluid, barbecue lighters, matches, charcoal, and any other accessories you'll be using. If you have a gas grill, lock it up, if possible. Otherwise, make sure children never have access to it.

CHAPTER 9

Advice for Caregivers

Y ou have done your homework educating yourself on what is and isn't safe for your kids, but what happens when you leave your child with a grandparent or a baby sitter? Don't assume your child's caregiver is as knowledgeable about safety issues and pitfalls as you are. Grandparents may need to brush up on a few topics; child-safety issues have changed greatly since they were young parents. Take the time to go over these simple safety guidelines with your sitter—grandparents included. Don't be afraid to give too much information or to offend a relative, friend, or professional with a list of safety tips—they'll understand that your child's safety is priority number one.

Give your sitter a tryout. No matter how well you know the person you have chosen to watch your child, you should always go through a "dry run" with her. Invite her to your house to play with your children while you're there. Feed your baby a bottle or your toddler dinner; this way she'll see what they eat and how the bottle or food is prepared. In addition, your children will get a chance to get used to her, your sitter will get used to your children and their environment, and you can answer any questions that may arise and point out any needs of your children, such as medications or special foods.

Write it down. Create a clearly written list of instructions for your sitter, including special food needs or medications your children should take. Review the list with your sitter during the dry run. Then, before you leave your children with the sitter, tell her that you have left the instructions posted in a prominent place, such as the refrigerator door.

Emergency phone numbers aren't enough. Chances are, you picked up your sitter and drove her to your home. She might not know your address and she probably hasn't memorized your phone number. If there is an emergency, the sitter should know how to direct emergency personnel. Make sure your sitter knows your street address, your last name, your home phone number, your cell phone number(s), and the name and number of the restaurant, place or friends' home you are visiting. Post a list of this information by every phone in the house.

Answering the phone is not job one. Make sure your sitter understands that answering the phone should never distract her from watching your children. If you want your sitter to answer the phone, give her guidelines for doing so and emphasize that it is fine to let it ring if necessary. Tell her never to walk away from the baby to answer the phone. If she is changing the baby, or if the baby is in the high chair or crawling around the house, let the answering machine pick up. She is a babysitter first and foremost, not a message center. A good strategy is to let the answering machine pick up all calls, but raise the volume so she can hear if you are calling in case of an emergency. Or tell her not to answer the phone, and get her cell phone number so you can contact her if necessary.

Bath duty is not for the sitter. Even if your little one ended dinner with more food in her hair than her mouth, don't let the sitter bathe your baby. Bath time is filled with a whole set of dangers that the sitter might not be used to handling. Instead of bathing your baby after feeding, tell the sitter to wipe the baby's face and hands with a clean washcloth and lukewarm water.

Explain how to feed your infant. You know to never prop up a bottle to feed your baby, and this is the type of advice you should pass on to your sitter. If your sitter is young, she may never have fed a baby before; if the grandparents are sitting, remember that they may not have fed a baby in quite some time. The dry run with the sitter is the time to make sure you are confident she is up to the task of giving your baby a bottle or feeding your infant or toddler.

Tips for Choosing a Baby Sitter

It goes without saying that you should be careful in choosing a person to take care of your children. Here are some guidelines compiled by Kyla Boyse, R.N., of the University of Michigan Health System, to help you choose a baby sitter you can trust.

- Enlist a trusted friend or family member if possible.
- Get recommendations from friends.
- Trade childcare with friends who have kids.
- Do not hire a sitter under age 12.

- Watch your child's reaction when you tell them a sitter they know is coming, and listen to what your child says about the sitter afterward.
- Meet the sitter in advance, and check references.
- Make sure the sitter knows CPR and first aid.
- Ask whether young sitters have taken a baby-sitting class from the American Red Cross. If not, encourage them to take it. If you have a sitter that you like, offer to pay for them to take the class.

Explain how to prepare a bottle. Whether your caregiver is giving your child previously pumped and stored breast milk or mixing formula, write down your instructions for the sitter and then review them with her. Have clean bottles and nipples ready. Explain that she must never use a microwave oven to heat a bottle. Instead, she should run the bottle under hot tap water until the contents are warm, then gently shake it to even out the temperature. She should test the milk or formula on the inside of her wrist to ensure it's no warmer than lukewarm before giving it to your baby.

List which foods are allowed and which are not. Don't just leave a list of foods your child cannot eat because of food allergies or intolerances. Make it easy for the sitter by listing foods your child is allowed to eat and likes. Be sure to have the approved foods on hand. If you have two or more children with different food needs, be sure to provide separate lists for each child. (See, "Watch for These Food-Allergy Symptoms," page 44.)

Point out choking hazards. Make sure your sitter knows about common choking hazards and that food must be cut into bite-sized pieces. A younger child may want what her older sibling is eating, and it is important for the sitter to know which foods present a choking hazard to younger kids. If this is the first time your sitter is feeding your child, you may even want to show her how big to make food pieces. If you didn't get around to a dry run with the sitter, it's a good idea to feed the baby with her the first time she watches your child. (See Chapter 5, "Food and Dining," page 39, for more on food allergies and food choking hazards.)

Emphasize that babies must sleep on their backs. Knowledge about safe sleep practices has improved over the years, so even older, experienced sitters or grandparents may not realize that they should place your baby on his back in the crib or bassinet. Tell the sitter to never place your baby on his stomach for sleeping, even for a nap. Doing so puts the baby at risk for sudden infant death syndrome (SIDS).

Is Your Child's Day Care Safe?

In a national study, Consumer Product Safety Commission staff visited child-care settings around the country and found that two-thirds of them had one or more potentially serious hazards. The following checklist will help ensure that you are leaving your young children in a safe place.

Cribs. Make sure cribs meet current national safety standards and are in good condition. Look for a certification safety seal. As at home, crib slats should be no more than $2\frac{3}{8}$ inches apart, and mattresses should fit snugly. This can prevent strangulation and suffocation associated with older cribs and with mattresses that are too small.

Bedding. Be sure that no pillows, soft bedding, or comforters are used where babies sleep. Babies should be put to sleep on their backs in a crib with a firm, flat mattress. This can help reduce sudden infant death syndrome (SIDS) and suffocation related to soft bedding.

Playground surfacing. Look for safe surfacing on outdoor playgrounds—at least 12 inches of wood chips, mulch, sand, or pea gravel, or mats made of safety-tested rubber or rubberlike materials. This helps protect against injuries from falls.

Playground maintenance. Check playground surfacing and equipment regularly to make sure they are maintained in good condition. This can help prevent injuries, especially from falls.

Safety gates. Be sure that safety gates are used to keep children away from potentially dangerous areas, especially stairs. Safety gates can protect against many hazards, including falls.

Window blinds and curtain cords. Be sure miniblinds and venetian blinds do not have looped cords. Check that vertical blinds, continuous-looped blinds and drapery cords have tension or tie-down devices to hold cords tight. Check that inner cord stops have been installed. These safety devices can prevent strangulation in loops of window blind and curtain cords.

Recalled products. Check that no recalled products are being used and that a current list of recalled children's products is readily visible. Recalled products pose a threat of injury or death.

Transportation. Children can die from heat or cold exposure if left in a vehicle, even in mild weather. If your child travels to day care by van or bus, make sure there is a procedure to ensure that no one is left in the vehicle. The driver or a helper should have a list of names that is checked off as each child gets on the bus and again when they get off, both going to the facility and coming home. When the vehicle arrives, the list should be double-checked by someone in the day-care facility. Parents of children who are not checked off should be called to ensure the child is indeed absent that day. In addition, the vehicle should be thoroughly checked when it arrives at day care and before it is parked for the night, including the floor and behind each seat, to make sure no child has fallen asleep and slipped out of sight.

✱ Advice for Caregivers

Show Caregivers How to Use Children's Products

You know how to use your high chair, stroller, and car seat, but your sitter or your child's grandpa might not. Show the caregiver how to properly strap your baby into the carriage, car seat and high chair, explain how these products work, and demonstrate the safety features that are integral to your child's well-being. Remember that improper use can lead to injury.

Guidelines for the high chair

• Make sure the chair is fully open and locked into place. Sometimes chairs look open, when actually they're not.
• Always use the safety-restraint straps. Even if the sitter is in the room, she must use the straps in the high chair.
• Allow no one to lean or climb on the high chair.
• Never put the high chair near a table, counter or wall. (A child will be able to push himself off from any accessible surface like this.)
• Never leave the room while a baby is in the high chair.

Guidelines for the stroller

• Always use the stroller's safety-restraint straps, even if your child will be in it for only a short time.
• Never leave a child unattended in a stroller. Children have died because they slipped feet-first through a leg opening and their head became entrapped between the seat and the restraint bar. This is a danger even for infants who are only a few weeks old. Be especially vigilant when using the stroller in the

fully reclined "carriage" position.
• Don't hang purses or shopping bags on the handles of the stroller; they can cause the stroller to tip. Even if the handles can manage the weight of bags, the stroller will tip when the sitter starts to remove your child. Also make your sitter aware of the weight limits in the basket and storage areas.

Guidelines for the car

• Install the car seat for your sitter every time. Don't expect her to know how to do it properly.
• Show your sitter how to secure your child in the car seat. Everything from the chest clip to the buckle must be used properly, be in the right position, and be fastened correctly. Demonstrate each detail for your sitter. (See "Installing Your Car Seat," page 116.)
• Some infant seats can be snapped into strollers. If your sitter will be taking the seat in and out of the car to use with the stroller, be sure to install an infant seat base in the car so she can just snap it in place.
• Your sitter should never give food or any other possible choking hazard to your infant or toddler while driving. She shouldn't try to pacify him with an object that could be dangerous in a crash, such as a heavy toy. Explain to the caregiver that in a crash whatever is in the vehicle can fly across the car striking your child. So everything inside the car must be safely stowed. That means all groceries and packages should be in the trunk.

Don't let your baby sleep on an adult bed. Your baby might fall asleep in the sitter's arms on the couch or in her grandpa's arms while he is resting on your bed. Whether you are leaving the little one at Grandma's house or with a sitter at home, make it clear that your baby is not to be put to sleep on an adult bed or any other place but her crib, play yard or bassinet. If you are leaving a play yard for your baby to sleep in, open and assemble it before you leave. Tell caregivers that if they use the changing station or a bassinet attachment on a play yard, it should be removed when the child is in the play yard, even when the child is sleeping.

Ban extra items from the crib. Make sure your caregiver knows what is allowed in your baby's sleep environment. The sitter or even a loving grandparent may want to add a favorite blanket or toy. But the safest crib has nothing in it but a mattress, a tightly fitting crib sheet and a baby. Be sure they know never to give your baby stuffed animals or toys with plastic buttons, eyes or noses that a baby can pull or choke on. Let them know that your baby needs to be on a firm, tight-fitting mattress so he can't slip into any cracks. (If you can fit more than two fingers between the side of the crib and the mattress, there is a dangerous gap.) Tell them never to add pillows, quilts, comforters and sheepskins to the bassinet or crib.

Explain about age-appropriate toys. If the sitter is watching more than one child, she should keep the older sibling's toys away from the younger child. Don't assume that grandparents or sitters understand the danger in sharing toys. Explain why the toys must be separated, and point out which ones are not to be used by the younger child. Just because you've put the toys away in a closet doesn't mean visitors in your home will know why they're out of sight. Make sure the sitter knows that small pieces can be choking hazards and sharp parts are dangerous, and that they should be removed from the play area.

Tell the sitter not leave anything on the floor that a child shouldn't put in his mouth. Even something simple, such as a charm on a necklace, can be dangerous. Caution her to keep all items that aren't designed for your baby, toddler or young child out of their reach.

Outline the general do's and don'ts in your home. In all likelihood, your sitter works for other families and the rules of each home are different. Explain the dangers you take for granted, like tipping furniture when a child climbs on bookcases, armoires, and TV-stands. (See "Use furniture restraints," p. 9.) If your child is using furniture to pull herself up, point out to the sitter which furniture is stable enough and which pieces to keep your child away from, such as armoires and TV stands. Also remind the sitter to keep a watchful eye on your little one at all times because your child might try things when you are away if the caregiver doesn't say no fast enough.

Over the River and Through the Woods

When visiting grandma and grandpa's house or anyone's house for that matter, follow these safety tips:
• Ask grandparents to remove potentially dangerous items from the floor as well as from areas your child may be using as a play space.
• Ask grandma to push small appliances back from the edges of the countertops, put away cords, remove tablecloths and use the back burners when she is cooking.
• Ask your hosts to put medicines, chemicals, cleaners, and any potentially hazardous items in a locked cabinet. Also ask them not to dispose of these items in a wastebasket, unless it is one that is kept in a locked cabinet.
• Ask grandma to be cognizant of everyday items she may typically leave on countertops or within a child's reach that could be hazardous to a child, such as food storage bags, aluminum foil, or plastic-wrap containers with a jagged edge, refrigerator magnets, and cleaning materials.
• As an extra precaution, you may want to safeguard grandma and grandpa's house by adding a few tip-resistant straps, table guards, outlet protectors, and corner cushions to furniture. (See Chapter 6, "Living Room and Dining Room," page 53.)
• Follow all the safety precautions you would follow for sitters at your own house. Be sure to provide grandparents with a safe sleeping environment for your child, such as a bassinet or play yard.

Prohibit sleeping on the job. There have been cases of serious injury to children when sitters napped when they napped. Be sure your sitter knows she needs to be fully attentive and to frequently check on your child during naptime.

Stow small appliances and cords. Before you leave the house, make sure that all small appliances are out of your children's reach. Be sure to stow any electrical cords that a child could use to pull an appliance onto him. For example, if you iron your shirt just before you go out, turning the iron off isn't enough. Make sure you unplug the iron *and* put it away. Caution the caregiver to make sure any appliance she uses is kept well out of your child's reach. Also remind her that she should never leave anything potentially harmful—such as a cup of coffee—on the edge of counters or tables.

Never leave the baby alone with an older sibling. The sitter may be tempted to ask a sibling for help, especially if the baby isn't used to the sitter. Remind her that she is in charge, not the sibling. The sibling might not know what to do if there's a problem.

Teach caregiver about vehicle dangers. Even if the baby sitter isn't driving your children, she may encounter your neighbor's car or someone pulling into your driveway. Your younger children should be in her arms or safely in the house in the crib or play yard when vehicles are pulling in and out of the driveway. Even older children should be brought to the side of the drive where they must hold the hand of an adult. In addition, she must walk all the way around her car before pulling out of your driveway. Explain that your children may try to run to greet her or say goodbye. She needs to be sure that your children—and others— are clearly not in the path of her car.

Is your sitter doubling as a cleaner? If your sitter is doing some cleaning, be sure she knows to keep any cleaning products out of your child's reach. She should clean only when your young child is napping in her crib. She can, however, multitask when caring for an older child, cleaning while keeping a watchful eye on him. Some children may want to help, but let your sitter know that your child should never be allowed to help if it involves using cleaning substances.

Does your sitter also have pet duty? Explain that pets and babies should be kept separate, especially when the child is asleep. (You can buy a crib tent that attaches securely to all standard cribs to keep pets out.) She should also keep the pet food and pet toys well out of reach of your infant or toddler. They can be a choking hazard.

CHAPTER 10

Holidays, Predators, and the Internet

S ometimes the most enjoyable events can carry hidden hazards. Rituals for Halloween and other holidays might seem innocuous enough—until a billowy costume or a small toy sends a child to the hospital. And as your child grows you won't be with him all the time, so he'll be vulnerable to adults who might do him harm both on the street and on the Internet. You and your child need to be armed with the crucial tips in this chapter to protect his safety, whether he's out trick-or-treating, walking home from school, or sitting quietly in your house surfing the Web.

Holiday Safety

Holidays are joyful celebrations—as long as you follow certain measures to keep your child safe. Keep these easy-to-remember tips in mind as you mark holidays and birthdays throughout the year.

Throw away wrapping paper. After opening gifts, toss all wrapping paper, strings, ribbon, and bows. A toddler can easily put a ribbon around her neck, a plastic bag over her head, or paper in her mouth while you are momentarily distracted.

Never throw wrapping paper into the fire. Don't let your children throw wrapping paper into the fire (and don't do it yourself). Fires started with wrapping paper burn rapidly and intensely, and they can create a flash fire. In addition, the inks used in wrapping paper may contain heavy-metal compounds and metallic materials, and even a small amount can pose risks when released into the air when the paper is burned.

Don't let your child touch holiday lights. In many cases, electrical cords contain lead, which can rub off on your hands and therefore shouldn't be handled by children. (In fact, wash your own hands thoroughly after you handle your light sets.) Make sure your lights sport the UL symbol with a holographic image. Those with the green holographic labels are for indoor use only; those with the red holographic label can be used indoors or outdoors.

Check all holiday lights, whether old or new. Don't use damaged lights. Check for loose connections and frayed or bare wires. Also look for broken or cracked sockets. Don't use lights for more than three 90-day seasons, and don't overload extension cords. Underwriters Laboratories recommends that you connect no more than three strings of push-in bulbs or a maximum of 50 screw-in bulbs together. Turn the lights off when you go to sleep.

Take care with candles. Place candles only in a nonflammable and heat-resistant container, at least a foot away from other materials. Keep them out of reach of children, definitely out of a child's room, and put matches where kids can't light candles after they've watched you do so. Never leave a burning candle unattended (especially with kids around) and put them out when you leave the room and before you go to sleep.

Check all toys. Don't let your toddler play with toys he receives as gifts unless you are sure they are age appropriate. Check them to make sure there aren't any small parts or pieces that can separate and become a choking hazard. Keep older kids' toys away from toddlers.

Accompany children under 12 when trick-or-treating. Pin a piece of paper with your child's name, address, and phone number inside a pocket in case she gets separated from you. Remind her where the number is located and be sure she has access to it. Older children should always trick-or-treat with a group.

Give cell phones to kids who are old enough to trick-or-treat on their own. Program all your phone numbers into it. Teach your child to only visit homes that are well lit and never to enter the home of a stranger, or even the home of an acquaintance that they haven't previously visited with you.

Make your trick-or-treater visible to all. Choose bright- and light-colored costumes and clothing. You want to be sure motorists can see your child. Buy reflective tape at your hardware or sporting goods store and attach it to your child's costume and candy sack. Give him a flashlight or glow stick to carry.

Look for flame-resistant costumes. Make sure all parts of your child's costume are flame resistant, including the mask and wig. Polyester and nylon are both flame-resistant materials but also look for the label "flame-resistant."

Buy costumes that fit. Don't purchase ones that are flimsy, billowing, too big, or drag on the ground. Your child will be doing a lot of walking and might climb steps as well. You want to be sure her costume isn't a tripping hazard and can't get caught in Halloween candles.

Avoid dangerous accessories. Make sure that no part of your child's costume—such as a sword, scepter, cane, or knife—is sharp. All should be made of a soft and flexible material. Some accessories can cause eye injuries and are best left at home. (Besides, you may find after visiting a few houses that you end up carrying your child's sword or other accessories.)

Check masks for proper visibility. Be sure your child tries on his mask before trick-or-treating. It should be secure and he should be able to breathe through it easily. The eyeholes should allow for full vision. Additional accessories such as scarves and hats should fit and be tied properly to avoid obstructing your child's eyes.

Your princess doesn't need heels. While high heels may make your child feel like a princess, keep them for dress up rather than for Halloween night. She should wear shoes that fit well and are sturdy and comfortable.

Bring extra treats with you. Bring candy that you have already examined for your child to eat. He shouldn't eat anything until you have had a chance to examine it for him.

Keep kids and costumes away from jack-o'-lanterns, whether indoors or out. Your child needs to know that the candle inside a pumpkin is not a toy and can possibly set a costume on fire. Don't leave a jack-o'-lantern that contains a burning candle unattended and and keep it away from curtains, furniture, and other items that could ignite.

Make your lawn and front steps safe for trick-or-treaters.
Remove obstacles and tripping hazards such as garden hoses and lawn ornaments. Sweep and remove leaves and make sure your front steps are well lit. Keep jack-o'-lanterns away from doorsteps and areas where children can brush up against them.

The costume your child wears is an important part of ensuring she has a safe and fun Halloween.

Do not obstruct vision: tie hat or scarves securely

Use cosmetics or wear properly fitted mask

Costumes, wigs and beards should be flame resistant

Carry flashlight to see and be seen

Decorate costume with reflective tape for better visibility

Well-fitting costumes and shoes prevent falling

Examine all treats before eating

Leave fireworks to the pros. Using fireworks on your own is both dangerous and, in many parts of the country, illegal. In 2006, fireworks caused 11 deaths and an estimated 9,000 injuries, with over a third of those injuries to children under 15, according the Consumer Product Safety Commission. If you insist on using fireworks, never allow young children to handle any of them, even sparklers, which burn very hot, can easily ignite clothing, and were responsible for an estimated 1,000 of those injuries, including 200 eye injuries. Keep fireworks well away from anything that could ignite and have a bucket of water on hand.

Personal Safety

Though you walk a fine line between arming your child with vital information and frightening her with scary scenarios, the bottom line is that you need to teach your child how to protect herself, particularly when she's not with you. The most important thing is communication. Honesty is the best policy. Tell your child that you do not want her to live a life that is fearful, but there are certain things we can all do to help ourselves so we can be in charge of our own lives. Here is essential information about personal safety that your child needs to know.

Help your preschooler memorize her address. He needs to have this information in case he gets separated from you in a public place. You can make up a song or a rhyme to make memorization easier.

Teach your child how and when to dial 911. By the time your child is 4 or 5 years old, she will understand the significance of dialing 911. Teach her why, when, and how this is done. Remember that learning your home number is good, but knowing 911 is better. It should be the first number called; your child will not always find someone at home.

Don't keep secrets. Teach your child early on that you must not have secrets from one another. Explain that there are bad secrets: Anything that another adult tells your child not to tell you is a bad secret. Make sure your child understands that he should always talk to you about anything that makes him uncomfortable.

Be aware of behavioral changes in your child. If something is wrong, your child may feel nervous coming to you for help or guidance. If you see changes in her behavior, try to be aware of not only what she is saying to you, but also what she might be holding back.

Strangers aren't the only ones who can cause harm. Many children are exploited or harmed by an acquaintance or family friend, rather than by a stranger; for example a coach, someone at the school or even a baby sitter or a member of the family. Teach your child to leave an uncomfortable situation as soon as possible—even if it involves someone he knows—and to tell you about it immediately.

Tell your child what an abductor might say, and what your child should do. For example, an abductor might tell her, "Mommy sent me." Explain that you would never send someone to pick her up from school or the playground without telling her. Or an abductor might ask if your child if she wants to see his kitten or dog or ask for help finding a lost pet. Explain that an adult should not ask a child for help and should not offer candy or toys to her. In each scenario, teach your child to say, "no," and quickly run to a safe place where there are other people, to an adult she knows, or to any authority figure like a teacher or police officer. She should tell this person what has happened. Also, make it clear to your child that she won't get in trouble for being impolite to an adult if she runs away because she feels threatened.

Tell your child who is allowed to pick her up from school or day-care. He must know who these people are and understand that you would never send a stranger to pick him up. He should never leave with someone he doesn't know. Ensure that workers at the school or day-care facility understand that your child is never to be released to anyone else unless you have informed them in advance.

Yell if there is danger. If, as mentioned, a person tries to cajole your child into coming with them with candy or other means, she should say no and run away. But the moment someone tries to grab a child, the child should yell as loudly as she can and get away as quickly as possible. She should yell a phrase that will make others quickly understand that a stranger is trying to abduct or harm her such as, "Someone is trying to take me away!" Simply yelling "no" won't alert others to danger or a possible abduction.

Use the buddy system. Children should always go places in groups or in pairs. There really is strength in numbers.

Teach your child to be aware of his surroundings. Make sure he knows who is around him as he walks home from school or a friend's house. If he feels someone is following him on foot or in a car, he should run quickly to a populated place, not a desolate or wooded area. He should run to a neighbor or friend's house or a store.

Show your child how to pull out of his jacket to escape a predator.

Head in the opposite direction of danger. Teach your child to run for help if she senses that someone is following her by car. If someone stops a vehicle to ask for directions, for help locating a pet, or for any other reason, your child should run away. She should never approach the car.

Teach your child how to get away. If someone tries to abduct him, he should immediately slip out of his jacket, shirt, or backpack and run away. If he can't escape he should wrap his arms and legs around something sturdy such as a fence or tree and yell, "A stranger is trying to take me away." If struggling with an abductor, strike him in a vulnerable place such as the face, throat, or groin and run away as quickly as possible.

Teach how to escape from an abductor's vehicle. If, despite all her efforts to escape, your child is pulled into a vehicle, she should do anything she can to get out. The first time the car stops, she should open the door, jump out, and run.

Seek a trustworthy person. Tell your child not to leave the premises if he gets lost or separated from you. Tell him to seek a trustworthy person for help; for example, he should go to a cashier if you're shopping at a store. He should never leave the store or get into a vehicle.

Teach your child to stick to you like glue. She should not run off to see a costumed character or even a friend or relative. You should always keep your child at your side, whether shopping or at a child's concert or event.

Keep a current color photo of your child with you. Be sure it has been taken in the past six months and clearly shows his head and shoulders. Know what clothing your child is wearing each day. You should be able to accurately describe your child and know his height, weight, hair color and length, eye color, scars, birthmarks, and any other identifying characteristics.

Don't advertise your child's name. Avoid putting her name on her clothing, bike, backpack, lunch box, playground toys, or anything she might carry with her. She will be confused—and vulnerable—if a stranger calls her by name.

Phone calls shouldn't get personal. Teach your child not to give any personal information to the person on the other end of the telephone line. If you have caller ID, tell him to answer the phone only if he recognizes the caller's phone number. If he does answer the phone tell him to take a message and say "My mom/dad can't come to the phone right now." He should not say "My mom and dad are at work and won't be home until 7."

Don't answer the door. Children under 12 should never open the door for anyone. Tell older kids that they can open the door for friends and family but no one else. Keep the doors locked and teach children under 12 that only you may answer the door. Set an example for him—and always look to see who is at the door before opening it. He needs to know that not every knock at the door needs to be answered.

Get an ID card for your child. Contact your local police and find out if your county issues an ID card that features your child's photo, fingerprints, and lists her physical characteristics; it can help the police if she gets abducted or goes missing. This service is often offered at safety or community events or through your local police department. You can also find kits online to make your own ID cards.

Internet Safety

These days, children learn computer skills at the same time they learn to read and write. While computers and educational Web sites are great learning tools, the Internet can also pose danger to your child's physical safety. Be sure to monitor the sites she visits and the amount of time she spends online. Follow the tips below and teach her that the stranger she meets on line is still the stranger you told her to avoid.

Look for signs your child may be at risk online. Later in this chapter you'll learn about software that can help you control how your child uses the Internet. But software is far from foolproof and nothing is as important as communicating with your child and physically monitoring his online activities. Here are signs that your child may be at risk online:

* Spends large amounts of time online, especially at night.
* Receives telephone calls from adults you don't know
* Receives long-distance calls or calls from numbers you don't recognize, or makes calls to these numbers.
* Receives gifts or letters from people you don't know.
* Quickly shuts off the computer monitor or switches Web sites when you enter the room.
* Uses an online account belonging to someone else.
* Becomes withdrawn from the family.

Avoid chat rooms. Most predators spend large amounts of time in chat rooms. They might pretend they are children or teenagers. If your child still visits chat rooms, she should never respond to messages or bulletin board postings that are suggestive, obscene, belligerent, or harassing. Some sites let you restrict who can contact your kids and whom they can contact. Also, there are sites for younger children that only allow your child to pick from a list of preselected questions and answers, thus making it impossible for a predator to ask them vital questions. Some sites set age limits that prohibit a child from joining until she is a particular age, but the sites have no way to enforce the age limit—a child can simply click yes when asked if she is old enough.

Never give out identifying information. While online, your child should never disclose his name, age, home address, school name, school team name, telephone number or any information that may identify who he is, where he lives or what activities he attends. He also should not call people he meets online. He may feel it's safer to make a call than to give out his number, but thanks to caller ID an offender can track his number. Some offenders even have 800 numbers or ask children to call them collect, so you may not identify a problem by checking your phone bill. Stress, too, that your child must never arrange a face-to-face meeting with someone he met online. Explain that this is just like getting into a stranger's car. By communicating with a stranger on the Internet he is allowing himself to get into a space that the stranger controls. Either way, your child is giving a stranger access to do him harm.

If you suspect your child is communicating with a predator online, talk to her about what is happening. Stop her from using the computer and get as many details as you can for the police. Then review what is on her computer. If she has received any sexually explicit images or she has been solicited online, contact your local or state law enforcement agency and the Federal Bureau of Investigation. You can find your local FBI office at *www.FBI.gov.* You can also contact the National Center for Missing and Exploited Children at *www.missingkids.com* or

Keep the Home Office Safe

Your home office is filled with stuff that could be dangerous to kids, so be sure you can lock the door to keep children out when you are not there. If you need to have the kids with you while you are working there, be sure to childproof the room with anti-tip devices, outlet covers and other methods discussed in Chapter 6, "Living Room and Dining Room," page 53. You might also keep a stash of items in your office that will occupy your child so you can work. This can be as simple as a box of crayons and a coloring book or some stickers and a sticker book. This entertainment box will keep him busy and away from sharp items on or in your desk. Here are other tips for a safe home office:

• Your desk should be off limits. Teach your child to stay away from your desk, and keep staplers and other sharp objects such as pushpins, pencils, paperclips, scissors, and letter openers well out of his reach. Lock up dangerous items when you are not using them.

• Teach your child never to touch equipment. Keep his hands away from printers, VCRs, DVD players and, shredders or anything else he could get his hand caught in. He may not know how to work this equipment, but he will copy the way you use it and could get hurt.

• Unplug your shredder after each use. Don't use it if your child is in the room. In addition, he should never be left unsupervised around a paper shredder.

703-274-3900 to report any incident. Or call their 24-hour CyberTipline at 800-THE-LOST (800-843-5678).

Monitor your child's phone calls as well as his computer. Online predators like to talk to children on the phone. Use Caller ID to determine who is calling your house. You can also contact your phone company to sign up for a service that lets you block your number from appearing on someone else's Caller ID. You can opt for a feature that rejects incoming calls that you block; it prevents people from calling your home anonymously. It's a good idea to monitor the phone numbers listed on your phone bill, but calls to toll-free numbers, such as 800 numbers, won't be listed. You can also purchase a device that lets you see the numbers dialed from your home phone. You will find these at some electronic stores.

Keep photographs off the Web. Never let your child upload pictures of herself onto the Internet or send them to people she doesn't know. Don't even allow photos of your home or neighborhood. A predator can get a lot of info from them. She should download pictures only from trusted friends and family. Pictures from unknown sources could contain sexually explicit images.

Remember that your child will use computers elsewhere. Your child will be exposed to the Internet at school, the library, or a friend's house. Find out what computer safeguards are employed by your child's school and other places where your child is using a computer. If you aren't comfortable with the safeguards that are in place, suggest new ones, such as parental controls or software that will let an adult choose which Web sites children can access. Confirm that there is a teacher in the room monitoring activities at the school or a parent in the room while they use the computer at a friend's house.

Talk to your child about potential online dangers. Tell her about possible online victimization and how to prevent it. Review the

Web sites she knows about, and tell her which sites she can visit. Remind her that whatever she is told online may or may not be true. Urge her to talk to you about anything she encounters that may make her uncomfortable. Let her know that someone may try to fool her into thinking she is being contacted by a friend or an acquaintance. She shouldn't communicate with someone unless it is someone she knows in person and you have approved,

Don't keep a computer in your child's bedroom. Keep it in a common room in the house. You should be able to see the screen when he is on the computer to monitor Web sites he is visiting and whom he is chatting with. Explain that you will be looking at his email, Instant Messaging and the chat rooms he visits. Tell your child that he should only respond to Instant Messages from someone he knows and you have approved. Show him how to block future messages from senders he doesn't know.

Use parental controls and blocking software. Software is available that allows you to log your child's activities, including those she has chatted with, Web sites she has visited and applications she has used. This will help alert you if you child is chatting with people you don't approve of, or visiting Web sites you don't want her to visit. The Windows and Macintosh operating systems include filters that you can use to prevent your child from accessing inappropriate sites. Your Internet service provider may also offer filters.

You should restrict access to your child's "spaces" and "blogs" to people she knows in person. This can be done by using the privacy settings when he is on social-networking sites. These features let you monitor some of your children's activities—but not all of them. You need to keep an eye on the screen as well.

CHAPTER 11

The Car

You face a twofold challenge when it comes to keeping your child safe in and around motor vehicles. Obviously, you need to make sure they have maximum protection in case of a crash—and that means choosing the right child restraint and using it correctly. For this reason, the first and biggest section of this chapter is devoted to choosing and installing car seats.

Perhaps less obviously, when it comes to cars, you also need to protect children from themselves. There are plenty of opportunities for an active, curious child to get into a world of trouble in and around a vehicle. So in the second part of this chapter you'll find more tips to keep your kids safe when they are in or around the car.

Child safety seats have reduced fatal injuries by 71 percent for infants (younger than 1 year old) and by 54 percent for toddlers (1 to 4 years old) in passenger cars, according to the National Highway Traffic Safety Administration (NHTSA). That's why correct choice and use of a car seat is one of the most important things you can do to keep your child safe.

But installing a car seat correctly can be tricky, especially if you have never done it before. In fact, some 80 percent of infant car seats are estimated to be installed or used incorrectly. To avoid becoming part of that statistic, you'll need to invest some time to learn about the different types of car seats and how to properly install and use the seat you buy. This knowledge could quite literally save your child's life some day.

Choosing a Car Seat

The first thing to know is that your child must face rearward until she is *at least* 1 year old and weighs at least 20 pounds. However, she can continue to sit facing the rear after these milestones depending on the car seat you buy. The American Academy of Pediatrics (AAP) recommends that you keep your child in the rear-facing position as long as possible but no longer than the maximum weight or height specified for the seat you own. At some point you'll switch to a front-facing seat, and later, a booster seat that works with the car's safety belt. Most states have specific age or weight and height requirements for when children are allowed to cease using child restraints but your child should remain in some kind of car seat until she is at least 4 feet 9 inches tall and can comfortably sit in a regular car seat using a safety belt. Here's a roadmap of your options:

You can start your newborn with a dedicated infant seat—the safest way to transport infants. Most infant seats are designed to hold children up to 22 pounds, although some will hold a child weighing up to 30 pounds.

Infant seats most often come with a detachable base that is installed in the vehicle's back seat, and all have a carrying handle. These let you move the carrier with your baby inside—especially handy if you want to let your baby continue snoozing when you take him out of the car. For those with a base, you need only snap the carrier in and out, which is much quicker and easier than installing a seat directly into the vehicle each time you use it. You can also purchase additional bases if you have more than one vehicle, and some seats snap into a stroller base for a complete travel system.

Carrying handle

Detachable base

Or start with a convertible seat.

Another option is to skip the infant seat and start out with a convertible seat that can be used in the rear-facing position for infants and then switched to the front-facing position at the appropriate weight and age. Most convertible seats allow a child to remain rear-facing longer, as recommended by the AAP, as they have higher weight and height limits, often 30 to 35 pounds, but lack the convenience of the carrier. A convertible seat can be reversed to allow a child to face the front, typically when she's around 40 pounds, though again some seats can accommodate more weight. Be sure to check the manual for your specific seat. A convertible seat must not be used once a child's head reaches the top of the seat or when they pass the weight limits of the harness. When the time comes, you'll need to switch to a booster seat that's used with the vehicle's safety belt.

A dedicated infant seat always faces rear.

Convertible seats start in the rear-facing position and then convert to front facing when your child gets older.

The next step can be a dedicated front-facing seat. This might be the next step if you started with a dedicated infant seat, and you can make that switch once your child reaches the rear-facing limit of the infant seat and is at least 1 year old. Dedicated front-

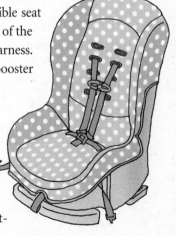

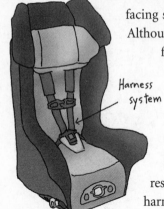

Harness system

A dedicated front-facing seat is one option for a child who outgrows a dedicated infant seat.

A combination seat has a removable harness so you can use it as a booster seat when your child gets bigger.

facing seats and convertible seats have built-in harnesses. Although most dedicated front-facing seats will hold a child from 20 pounds to approximately 40 pounds, some will hold a heavier child in a five-point harness.

Or try a combination child restraint. Another option after your child has outgrown his infant seat is to move your little one into a harness/booster combo known as a combination child restraint. These forward-facing seats have a removable harness that's designed to be used for a specified weight range—usually 20 to 40 pounds. Then you can remove the harness and use the seat as a belt-positioning booster with the car's seat belt.

Then move on to the booster. A booster seat raises your child enough so you can safely secure her with a safety belt. Belt-positioning boosters have a path that helps position the belt correctly across the child's chest and hips. You can get a backless booster or a high-back booster. The high-back models are best for vehicles that don't have head restraints built into the back seat. Some high-back belt-positioning boosters can convert to a backless one.

Your booster seat will have a minimum weight requirement—usually 30 to 40 pounds—for one, but weight is not the only determination of when your child is ready. He must be tall enough so that the shoulder belt does not fall across his neck; the belt must fit snugly across the chest and collarbone; and the lap portion must fit low enough across the top of his thighs that he can bend his knees comfortably.

As mentioned, you'll need to use the booster seat

with a safety belt until your child can comfortably ride in the vehicle seat with her back against the seatback, knees folded at the front of the seat cushion and with the belts crossing at her chest and upper thighs, typically when a child is around 4 feet 9 inches tall. Check your state laws for requirements on weight and age as well.

It's the law. All 50 states have child-passenger safety laws requiring the use of an appropriate restraint device. Most have laws setting a minimum age for use of an appropriate restraint device or booster for children who have outgrown their child safety seat but are too small for a safety belt. Kids typically reach this stage by age 4. Even when your child passes the age requirement for a safety seat or booster, you should continue to restrain him in the safest way possible for his height and weight—in the back seat until age 13.

All boosters must be used with your car's lap and shoulder belt. A high-back booster is a good idea for vehicles that don't have headrests in the back seat.

Buy your infant seat before your baby is born, so you can install it before you take your newborn home from the hospital. Try installing the seat well in advance of your due date so you can return it if it doesn't fit in your car.

Test fit that second seat. When it's time for Junior's second car seat, take him along when you shop so you can place him in various seats to see how he fits before you lay down your cash. If there isn't a floor model to try, don't hesitate to ask a salesperson to take a seat out of the box. You'll also want to try fitting the seat into your car before you make your final decision to be sure you have the best possible fit. Many retailers will let you

113

Getting to Know Your Car Seat

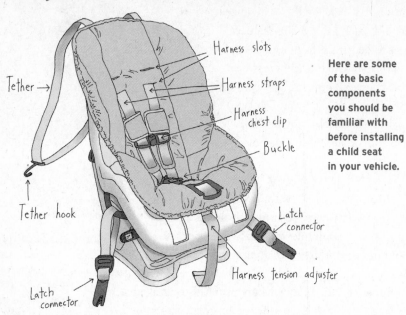

Tether →

Harness slots

Harness straps

Harness chest clip

Buckle

Tether hook

Latch connector

Latch connector

Harness tension adjuster

Here are some of the basic components you should be familiar with before installing a child seat in your vehicle.

To ensure that your car seat is properly installed, and to make the process as quick and easy as possible, it's really helpful to be familiar with the components. In addition to reading the following information, be sure to carefully read your instruction manual and the car-seat installation section of your vehicle owner's manual. Also study the labels on the seat itself. Be sure to keep your car-seat manual so you can refer to it when reinstalling the seat, changing it to another position, or moving it to another car. All seats have a place to store the manual.

Harness straps. These help restrain your child in the seat, just as a safety belt holds you in your seat.

Harness slots. The harness straps fit through these slots. The height of the straps must be adjusted to fit your child. When your baby is facing the rear, the harness should be threaded through the slots at or just below your baby's shoulders. When she's facing

forward, the harness should be threaded through slots at or slightly above her shoulders.

Harness tension adjuster. Used to loosen or tighten the harness system, this is located on the front of some seats and on the back of others. Harnesses should be tight enough around the child so you can't easily pinch a portion of the strap between your fingers, and you can't fit more than one finger comfortably between the child's collarbone and the harness.

Harness adjuster. Found on the back of the seat, this mechanism allows you to change the height of the harness straps or remove them to clean the straps and the seat cover. The method of adjusting a harness differs. Some seats have a device that allows adjustment without removing or rethreading the straps. On others you have to remove and rethread the harness, which is attached with a plate or clip at the back of the seat.

Harness chest clip. This helps correctly position the harness straps. Once your child is buckled in, the chest clip should be at armpit level.

Buckle. Located between your child's legs, the buckle fastens the harness.

LATCH connectors. LATCH stands for lower anchors and tethers for children and offers an alternative to the safety belts for installing child seats. The anchors are located in your car's seat back in the crease where the seat back and bottom meet. There is also an upper anchorage that allows the seat to be secured to the vehicle using the tether strap at the top of the child seat. The top tether anchor has been required in vehicles manufactured since Sept. 1, 2000. All vehicles manufactured after Sept. 1, 2002 have been required to have lower anchors in at least two rear seating positions and at least one top tether.

Belt path. Your child restraint seat has a path that the vehicle safety belt must pass through to correctly install the seat if you are using the car's safety belt instead of the LATCH system. Convertible seats have two paths, one for rear-facing installation and one for front-facing installation.

Tether. Convertible, front-facing, and combination seats have a tether at the top that connects to an anchor behind the vehicle's seat. Tether attachment is important to reduce the forward motion of a child's head during a crash.

Base-angle adjuster: This device is found on dedicated infant seats and convertible seats that can be used in a rear-facing position. It helps position the seat at the correct angle of about 45 degrees. Check your safety seat's manual for specific directions on using the adjuster. Most infant seats have a "foot" that can be dropped down from the base of your seat and adjusted to accommodate different seat angles. Turning a handle, pushing a button, twisting a knob, or moving some other device alters the position of this foot.

Level indicator: This helps you determine whether a rear-facing seat is at the correct angle. There are many types of level indicators. Your owner's manual will explain the one on your seat and where it is located.

Pool noodle or rolled towel: If your seat doesn't have a "foot" that can be adjusted to achieve the correct angle, you might need to use a pool noodle or rolled towel to do the job. Check your safety-seat instructions to see whether the manufacturer recommends using a positioning device to achieve this angle, which products can be used, and how to use them.

try one before buying it, but if not be sure of their return policy in the event the seat doesn't fit.

Check the expiration date. All child restraint seats have an expiration date, usually six years from the date of manufacture. It will be marked somewhere on the seat, often on the bottom. Check this date if you are dusting off an older sibling's seat for use with a new baby.

It's best to buy new. Usually, there is no way to determine the history of a used seat, including whether it was in a crash or is missing a part. The seat could be missing important labels or instructions, and it won't have a registration card. If the manufacturer doesn't have you registered as the owner, you won't be notified if the seat is recalled. It may also have reached its expiration date. Unless you can determine all of this information, don't consider buying a used seat.

Register your child safety seat by sending in the registration card or, if available, registering online with the manufacturer. Registering your seat is the only way to ensure you will be notified in the event of a recall. In addition, be vigilant about checking to find out if your seat has been recalled by going to the government's recall Web site at *www.recalls.gov* or NHTSA's Web site at *www.nhtsa.dot.gov*.

In the event of a crash, discontinue use of your child safety seat and purchase a new one. Even if the seat looks fine there could be internal damage that might prevent it from performing correctly and safely in another crash. You will also need to replace the vehicle belts that were in use during a crash.

Installing Your Car Seat

Here you will find some general guidelines and things to watch out for when you install your child car seat. However, installation procedures vary from model to model, so you'll need to read and follow the instructions in the manual that came with your particular seat and your car. If you are at all unsure about whether you are installing your car seat correctly, you can have your installation checked by a certified child-passenger safety seat technician. To find one in your area, call your local police department or go to *www.nhtsa.gov/cps/cpsfitting*.

Remember, the car seat always goes in the back seat, the only safe place for your child until he turns 13 years old. Never place a child seat behind an air bag. If the seat will fit correctly and securely in the middle of the back seat and there is room for other passengers, that's the best choice.

Never shove the back of the car's front seat up against the back of a rear-facing child seat. It's best if the front seat doesn't touch the child seat at all, but its OK for them to touch lightly if you need the leg room to drive.

Get the right angle. Your rear-facing infant car seat should be tilted just enough for your baby to lay her head back comfortably, typically around 45 degrees. If she's sitting too upright, her head could drop forward, cutting off her airway. However, if her head is too far back you'll create a risk of absorbing the forces of a crash in the head, neck and shoulders. As your baby develops more neck strength and is able to hold her head up, the seat can be in a more upright position; if her head falls forward, you'll know the seat is not tilted back enough.

Check the owner's manual for your infant seat for information about correct tilt angles and how to achieve them. Most rear-facing and convertible seats have some kind of built-in leveling device, and most also have a level indicator. Sometimes the indicator has a device such as a bubble, ball or color that tells you when the seat is at the correct angle. In other cases there is a reference line etched or pasted onto the seat. Be sure your vehicle is on a level surface when you use the indicator.

If you can't achieve the correct angle with the leveling device on your seat, or if your seat doesn't have a built-in leveling device, you can use a rolled towel or pool noodle at the crease of the vehicle seat to help position the infant seat at the correct angle.

Hands off the switches! If you place your seat next to a window, make sure your child doesn't play with door locks and windows. Teach your child not to touch the window and door-lock buttons and not to stick his hands outside of the window. If you have childproof locks, make sure they are engaged.

Securing with a Vehicle Safety Belt or LATCH

You'll have to decide whether LATCH anchors or the vehicle safety belt is the best way to install a child seat in your particular vehicle. For example, some LATCH anchors are so deep in the seat crease that you will find it easier to use the safety belt. Some safety belts require a locking clip that makes seat installation more difficult. Try both methods to see which works best and decide which will be easiest should you have to take the seat out. LATCH anchors are typically designed to hold a child up to 48 pounds (check your owner's manual in case your car has different weight limits), so once your child reaches this weight, the seat must be fastened using the safety belt.

Read car and seat manuals. There are several types of vehicle safety belts. Consult your vehicle owner's manual to find out which type you have. Then read the instructions that came with the child car seat to learn how to install it with the safety belt you have.

Get a tight installation. Whether you are using the vehicle safety belt or the LATCH system, it's important to secure the car seat as tightly as possible. Use your weight to push the child seat into the vehicle's seat (you might want to use your knee) while taking up the slack in the LATCH strap or safety belt. Once installed, the seat base or seat should have no more than 1 inch of movement either side to side or forward and back.

Stow the vehicle's safety belt. If you use LATCH, lock the car's safety belt behind the seat or secure it out of the way so that your child cannot reach it and become entangled.

Use the correct anchors. Be sure that each car-seat LATCH connector is attached to its own vehicle anchor on each side of the seat. The instruction manual for the car should indicate these locations (some have stickers identifying them). If you are installing two child seats in your vehicle, be sure they are not connected to the same anchors.

Be sure to tether front-facing seats. When using any seat in the front-facing position, always use the tether at top. Tethering the seat provides extra protection by increasing stability, providing a more secure installation, and limiting the movement of a child's head in a crash. When installing the seat, be sure to read the instructions regarding the tether, and connect the child seat to the tether anchor in your vehicle. Your vehicle owner's manual gives the tether anchor locations. If you have an older vehicle you can retrofit an anchor for tethering.

Detach the base before installing infant seats. The detachable bases on infant seats are a real convenience; snapping the seat into place is a lot easier than wrestling with safety belts or LATCH connectors each time. Detach the base from the seat before installing it in the car and then install the seat. Check the base before each use to ensure it is still secure. Then snap the seat into place. Listen for a click or other sound indicating the seat is locked to the base.

Securing Your Child in the Car Seat

Dress your little one lightly for a car ride. Don't put him in a car seat while he is wearing a heavy winter coat or layers of clothing. The clothing can compress during a crash, actually making the harness loose. On cold days, warm up the car, then carry out your little one wrapped in a warm blanket. Unwrap your baby, secure him in the car seat and then, if necessary, place a blanket over the seat and harness system.

Position harness straps properly. When your child is facing the rear, the harness straps should be at shoulder level or slightly below. The harness chest clip should be placed at the same level as his armpits. This keeps the harness straps positioned properly. Check your car seat manual to find out precisely how to secure the harness.

Your doctor may recommend a rolled towel or a towel on each side of your infant's head to support his neck. Be sure the towel does not inhibit the harness system of the seat.

Harness straps should fit snugly. Make sure the straps lie in a straight line, are not twisted, and don't sag. You should not be able to easily pinch any fabric along the length of the straps when they are tight.

When your child is facing front, the harness straps should be at or slightly above her shoulders. The convertible seat may be slightly reclined or upright when facing front. Also be aware that many convertible seats have a front-facing safety-belt path that differs from the rear-facing path.

When your child is in a booster seat be sure the vehicle safety belt fits properly. It must cross his chest, never lie across his neck. The lap portion of the belt should fit low and snug across the thighs; it should never cross the abdomen. When the belt is properly fitted, your child will be able to sit all the way back in her seat with her legs bent at the knees.

Only use a lap/shoulder belt combination with your booster seat, never a lap belt alone. A child can be seriously injured with only a lap belt.

Make sure the shoulder belt stays in place. If your child becomes fidgety or uncomfortable in a booster seat, she might try to place the shoulder portion of the belt behind her or under her armpits. Don't allow these dangerous positions.

Harness strap at or slightly above shoulders

Chest clips at armpit height

This drawing shows the correct positions for the chest clip and harness strap.

Minimize the slack. If the safety-belt system in your vehicle allows it, reduce the slack when installing your child in a belt-positioning booster by pulling the safety belt all the way out so that it locks when you release it. Your child will not be able to pull any slack from the belt once it's locked.

Integrated seats make life easier. Some vehicles have integrated safety seats with a five-point harness for securing your child directly into the vehicle. Check your vehicle instructions for the height and weight restrictions as well as the appropriate use for this type of seat. Be sure the harness and chest clip are positioned properly and that you have a proper and secure fit.

Position the safety belt properly. When your child is ready to use a safety belt, it should have the same fit as it did when he was in his booster seat. The shoulder belt should cross his chest and never lie across his neck. The lap portion should fit low and snug across the thighs, and never cross his abdomen. When the belt is properly fitted, your child will be able to sit comfortably all the way back in the vehicle seat with his knees comfortably bent across the vehicle's cushion.

Never use aftermarket products with your child-restraint seat. Use only the components that came with your car seat or are recommended by the manufacturer for your seat. Aftermarket products have not been tested with your child safety seat and so might not be safe.

Give soft toys only. Remember that anything you give to a child could become a projectile in a crash. So give him only soft toys to play with while traveling in the car. And as you know, anything you give a young child will probably end up in his mouth. It's especially important to avoid choking hazards while driving since you won't be able to grab objects away from your infant.

Check your exhaust system. Carbon monoxide poisoning most often happens in the garage, but it is also a hazard while you are driving if your exhaust system leaks. Have it checked during regular service or if you hear any change in exhaust noise, especially during cold weather when the engine uses more fuel to warm up and run.

Check all blind zones. No matter the size of your vehicle, there are blind zones that will hide the presence of a child behind, next to, or even in front of it. Some blind zones are bigger than the average driveway. Walk all the way around your vehicle before moving it to make sure no child is in any of your blind zones.

Keep in mind, though, that by the time you get in the car and begin to move it, a child could have easily arrived and might not be visible in the rearview mirror. So make sure you know exactly where your children are when you're about to drive away. Be especially careful when leaving a parking spot at another family's home, a day-care center, a school, or any other place where children might be around.

Consider a rearview camera. If you're in the market for a new car, consider buying one that comes with a rearview camera to alert you to objects behind it. There are also backup sensor systems that provide an audible warning, but CONSUMER REPORTS has found that these are handy for parking but are not reliable as a safety system. Even with a rearview camera, be sure to check behind the vehicle and look in your rearview mirror and then over your shoulder when backing up. If your vehicle doesn't have a rearview camera, you can have one retrofitted.

Take care when closing car windows. Be sure to check that all passengers have their arms, hands and fingers out of the way. Some cars have sensors that will stop a window from moving upward if anything is in the way. If you want to test whether your car has this feature, use a water bottle. Don't test with your finger—car windows can cut through a finger or severely damage a limb. Window sensors typically can't be retrofitted, so find out when you purchase your car whether it has this feature. Be aware that some models have these sensors for the driver's windows but not in the rear, where your children should be riding.

Janette Fennell, founder of Kids and Cars, a national non-profit group that works to improve child safety around cars, suggests, "You may want to institute a rule: Everyone needs to sit on their hands before windows are rolled up."

Never leave your child alone in a car, even for a quick errand, such as running in to pay for gas. Leaving a child in a car puts her at risk

How Big Is Your Blind Zone?

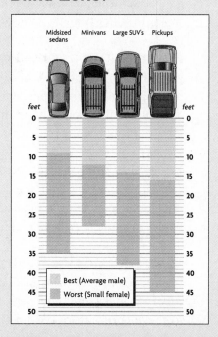

To help consumers understand how large some blind spots are, CONSUMER REPORTS measured the blind spots of a number of popular models. The results for both an average-height driver (5 feet 8 inches) and a shorter driver (5 feet 1 inch) are shown here.

for abduction, hyperthermia (overheating), or hypothermia (dangerously low body temperature). Other dangers include knocking a vehicle into gear, power window or safety-belt strangulation, carbon-monoxide poisoning or falling from the vehicle.

No napping in a parked car. Never leave your child napping in your car, even at a private home or in your garage. A car's windows trap heat. Your child's body temperature can rise three to five times faster than an adult's, quickly putting him in danger even in mild weather. Never leave your child unattended in a vehicle, even with the windows down.

Keep kids out of unattended cars. Never leave your keys in a vehicle, let your child sit in the driver's seat of your car, or let your children inside your car without an adult. In some vehicles your child might be able to set the vehicle into motion by simply moving the gearshift.

Show your kids the trunk release. Your child should know how to escape from a car trunk in case the lid is ever closed with him inside. All cars manufactured after Sept. 1, 2001 (model year 2002) are required to be equipped with a release mechanism inside the trunk to make it possible for a person trapped inside to escape. The mechanism can be a lighted or glowing latch, or it can be one that detects the presence of a human in the trunk and automatically unlatches the lid. Check the owner's manual and then show your kids how to do it.

Test garage-door openers. Place a 2-inch-high block of wood on the floor in the door's path. If the door doesn't reverse direction and go up when it touches the block, don't use the garage-door opener. In addition to reversing when they come in contact with something, new opener systems are equipped with optical sensors that prevent the garage door from closing if a child or anything else gets in the way. Even if these safety devices work perfectly, keep your child away from the garage door when it is opening and closing, because no device is foolproof.

CHAPTER 12

On the Go

Whether running errands, taking children to school, birthday parties, the playground, play dates, or simply enjoying activities together, you never seem to stop moving—and you have a little one moving right along with you. If you aren't in the car, you and your child are walking, enjoying a stroller ride, or cycling together. Whatever the activity, you'll need to practice safety on the go. According to the National Highway Traffic Safety Administration (NHTSA), injuries associated with bicycles send more 5 to 14 year olds to the emergency room than any other sport. Pedestrian safety is critical, too: NHTSA says that about one-third of the children ages 5 to 9 who are killed by motor vehicles are pedestrians. To prevent these and other on-the-go injuries, keep the following tips in mind as you head out the door.

Stash age-appropriate toys in your baby's diaper bag to give your baby when you're changing a diaper and on the move. A toy can pacify a squirmy baby, making it easier to prevent him from rolling or trying to climb off the changing table.

You can rotate toys so you aren't always giving him the same one, or you can surprise him with his favorite. Always use the safety strap on a changing table.

Beware of old strollers. It's best to purchase a new stroller that comes with a Juvenile Products Manufacturers Association (JPMA) certification program sticker on the carton or frame showing that it meets the ASTM International voluntary standard for strollers. ASTM published a new standard for strollers in early 2007, so models made before then may not meet current standards. Be wary of hand-me-down strollers, ones you used for a previous child, and those you might find at yard sales, on eBay, or on Craigslist. Check *www.cpsc.gov* to make sure any stroller you're considering or using has not been recalled.

Use the harness to restrain your child in a stroller. Don't place heavy objects on the stroller tray or hang them from the handles. And don't overload the storage basket.

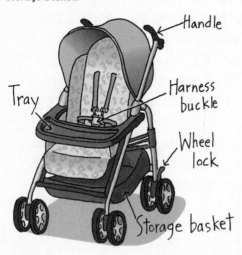

Handle

Harness buckle

Wheel lock

Tray

Storage basket

Always use the harness. Strap your child into her stroller even if she's squirmy and the trip is short. If the stroller hits an unexpected bump or if it tips, you want to be sure she is safely buckled in. Without a harness she could wriggle out of the stroller, or she could slip down and become trapped between the seat and the tray. Make sure the restraints work properly and the stitching is secure.

Make sure your baby sleeps safely in his stroller. Your child will undoubtedly fall asleep in the stroller. If the stroller seat is in the reclined "carriage" position, be sure that you can close off the leg openings to prevent the child from slipping through. If your stroller does not have this feature, keep the backrest upright.

Always use stroller brakes. Make it a habit: If your hands are off the stroller the brakes are on. It's the only way to make sure you have the stroller under your control.

Never leave your child unattended in a stroller, even if your child is asleep, buckled in and the brakes are locked. He may wake up, become upset, and try to climb out of the stroller, causing it to tip. Or he may slip through a leg hole and become trapped.

Know the weight limit. Stop using a stroller when your child has reached the weight limit recommended by the manufacturer. You'll find it in the owner's manual.

Don't hang heavy objects on stroller handles. Weighty grocery bags or diaper bags can cause the stroller to tip, especially as you're going over a curb or a bump. Also note that stroller storage areas have weight limits, which you'll find in the owner's manual.

Don't overload the tray. Don't put heavy objects or hot drinks on the stroller tray. And don't lift the stroller by the tray.

Don't let your child climb on the stroller or use it as a toy. Your children need to know that the stroller is not something to play with. Climbing on it can cause it to tip or trap a child. If your little one thinks pushing a stroller is fun, get him a toy version.

Age Guidelines for Ride-On Toys

These Consumer Product Safety Commission (CPSC) guidelines can help you decide which ride-on toys are appropriate for your child. Since children grow and develop physical strength and coordination at different rates, use these guidelines to inform your own best judgment.

• Be sure your child has a safe riding area, where he can navigate without the risk of going into traffic, down steep hills, on steps, or into driveways. If that's not possible, allow him to use a riding toy only inside or for trips to the park, where there are pathways he must use for riding.
• From 12 to 18 months, children who have learned to walk steadily can use ride-on toys, preferably with four wheels for stability, that they straddle and propel with their feet. Wheels should be spaced far enough apart to make the toy stable, but not so far apart that they make it difficult for a child to swing a leg over the seat. The toys should be low to the ground for easy mounting and dismounting. Children's feet should be flat on the floor when they are seated. Recessed wheels make it easier for a child to push along without catching their feet on the wheels.
• From 19 to 23 months, children can operate ride-on toys they sit inside and propel with their feet. Children of this age are unlikely to have steering skills needed to avoid obstacles and hazards, so they should be supervised.
• At 2 years, children like realistic-looking vehicles, such as pretend fire engines. They can ride a toy that moves when they bounce up and down in the seat. Two-year-olds are learning to pedal and may start

Keep your child away from the stroller when you're folding it. Her fingers and hands can get caught.

There's no rush to ride. Kids develop the coordination and the desire to ride a bike without training wheels at different times, so there's no need to push your child to ride just because other kids her age are riding or she's reached the "appropriate" age. If she doesn't show interest or is having a difficult time when trying to learn, no big deal, just try again in a month or two.

Buy a bike that fits. Your youngster can't ride safely and comfortably unless he has a bike that fits. Bikes that are too big are especially dangerous, using tricycles with pedals—especially as they get closer to 3. You'll need to stay close and be watchful, since kids of this age still don't have the steering and pedaling skills needed to avoid obstacles.

• At 3 years, many children have developed the ability to use three-wheeled scooters, but they may not have developed the balance required to operate two-wheeled scooters and bicycles. They can use a small bicycle with training wheels and footbrakes. Children at this age can steer a slow-moving battery-operated vehicle.

• At 4 through 5 years, children begin to show an interest in skateboards. They can use battery-operated vehicles. Most children by the age of 5 have the balance and coordination to use two-wheeled scooters and bicycles without training wheels. But they might not understand the dangers of riding in areas with cars, and are at very high risk of falling and injuring themselves. Adult supervision is a must.

• At 6 through 8 years, most children have the physical ability to ride a bicycle without training wheels and have developed the coordination to use hand brakes. They can operate slow-moving motorized vehicles, particularly those with four wheels.

• At 9 through 12 years, most children are very capable bicycle and scooter riders, and they can use bicycles with hand gears for different speeds. They can usually operate a motorized wheeled vehicle that does not exceed 10 mph and has gear shifting. Faster-moving motorized bicycles and scooters are generally not appropriate even for 12-year-olds because of the difficulty of balancing and steering while moving.

so you don't want to buy one for him to "grow into." And while it would be fun to surprise him with a new bike, it's much more important to take him to the store to pick out one that fits properly. Here's more advice from the American Academy of Pediatrics:

✳ Make sure your child can rest the balls of both feet on the ground when he sits on the bike with his hands on the handlebars.

✳ Straddling the center bar, your child should be able to stand with both feet flat on the ground with about 1 inch of clearance between his crotch and the bar.

✳ When buying a bike with hand brakes for an older child, make sure he can comfortably grasp them and apply sufficient pressure to stop the bike.

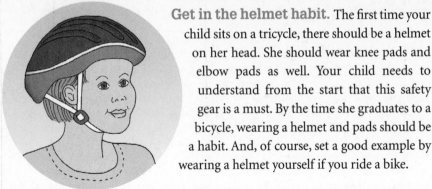

Get in the helmet habit. The first time your child sits on a tricycle, there should be a helmet on her head. She should wear knee pads and elbow pads as well. Your child needs to understand from the start that this safety gear is a must. By the time she graduates to a bicycle, wearing a helmet and pads should be a habit. And, of course, set a good example by wearing a helmet yourself if you ride a bike.

A bike helmet should be worn level, as shown here, not pushed back. The side straps should form a "V" beneath the ears.

Check the label. Don't buy a new helmet unless it has a label indicating that it meets safety standards set by the U.S. Consumer Product Safety Commission (CPSC). Don't use an old helmet unless it has a label stating that it meets one of the voluntary safety standards from ASTM International, the Snell Memorial Foundation, or the American National Standards Institute (ANSI). And never use an old helmet unless you are sure it has never been in an accident.

Fit is foremost. A helmet won't do much good if it doesn't fit well. A bike store is the best place to buy one because a knowledgeable store employee can help you find one that fits your child properly. Here are some guidelines:

* Use the appropriate foam pads and rear stabilizer or the helmet's fit system to create a snug (but not tight) fit when you place the helmet level on your child's head.

* With the chin strap buckled and all other straps tight, push up firmly on the helmet's front edge. If the helmet moves enough to expose the forehead, shorten the front straps, then tighten the chin strap enough so that the helmet pulls down when your child open his mouth. Repeat as necessary.

* Grasp the helmet by its rear edge and tilt forward. If it moves enough to cover your child's eyes, shorten the back straps (but leave the

front straps alone). Repeat as necessary.

* If you can't get a satisfactory fit, choose another model.

Remove the helmet after riding. Don't allow your child to wear his helmet when he's playing on playground equipment or climbing trees. The strap can snag and strangle him. Once he is done riding his bicycle, he should remove his helmet.

Replace the helmet after a crash. Even if the helmet appears unscratched, it may have been damaged internally. Buy a new one after a crash to ensure that your child gets the best protection.

Don't carry infants on a bicycle. Any child riding on a bicycle should wear a helmet, but helmets aren't made for children under the age of 1 year. For this reason, you shouldn't carry a child in a bicycle-mounted child seat, a trailer, or other carrier until she is old enough to wear a helmet. Even as your little one becomes a toddler, her neck muscles may not be able to support the weight of a helmet. You may even want to wait until your child is 2 years old. If you are not sure, take your child and the helmet to your family doctor or pediatrician for advice.

Learn to brake first. Your child needs to know how to use the brakes on his bicycle before learning anything else. Show him how to stop by holding onto the bike and gently moving forward as your child uses the brakes until you are confident he knows how.

Bright is best. Your child and anyone riding with her should wear bright colors or reflective stripes on their clothing or sneakers. Don't go biking at dusk or at night.

Watch for obstacles. Keep an eye out for obstacles in your little rider's path that could cause her to swerve, tip, or make a sudden turn. She should also learn to watch for obstacles herself.

Be sure the bike is working properly. Check your child's bicycle regularly. Does the seat still fit him correctly? Are the brakes in good shape? Are the wheels fastened securely?

Help with balancing. When the training wheels come off, you need to teach your child how to balance on a two-wheeler. The Bicycle Helmet Safety Institute (BHSI) recommends that you run alongside the bike, holding it by the seat with one hand and keeping the other on the handlebars to keep the bike upright.

Teach the rules of safe sidewalk riding. In general, the safest place to ride a bicycle is in the street, where bicycles are expected to follow the same rules of the road and ride in the same direction as motor vehicles. But children under 10 aren't mature enough to make the decisions necessary to negotiate traffic on their own and are better off riding on the sidewalk. Call your town hall to make sure sidewalk riding is allowed. If it is, teach your children the following guidelines from NHTSA:

* Watch for vehicles coming out of or turning into driveways.
* Stop at corners of sidewalks and streets to look for cars and to make sure the drivers see you before crossing.
* Enter a street at a corner and not between parked cars. Alert pedestrians that you are near by saying, "Excuse me," or "Passing on your left," or by using a bell or horn.

Demonstrate the rules of the road. When your child starts riding in the street it's a good idea to accompany her until you are sure she understands the rules of the road. Show your child how you obey traffic lights and stop signs, whether or not you see vehicles in the immediate vicinity. Demonstrate how to look left, right, and left again when crossing a street, and walk your bicycle through busy intersections.

Remember blind zones. Your child might see a vehicle, but the person driving it might not see your child. All vehicles have blind zones that prevent the driver from seeing a child walking or riding a bicycle. Teach your child that drivers might not see him and that he has to take precautions. He should never cut in front of or behind a vehicle—moving or stopped. When crossing in front of a car stopped at an intersection, he should get off his bike, make sure the driver sees him, and then walk.

The right side is correct. Your child should ride with traffic on the right-hand side of the road.

Turn correctly. Your child should learn to turn her head and look over her shoulder before turning, changing lanes, or swerving. She should not ride on the street on her own until she has mastered this skill.

Don't just follow. Your child needs to learn to obey the rules of the road whether or not the rider in front of him is doing so.

Make sure your child is wearing a helmet, knee pads and elbow pads when riding a scooter.

Use scooters with caution. Scooters send thousands of children to emergency rooms each year. Always closely supervise children who are 8 years old or younger when they ride a scooter, and teach them these rules for safe scooting:

* Always wear a certified bike helmet, knee pads, and elbow pads.
* Stop riding your scooter as soon as it starts to get dark.
* Always ride your scooter on the sidewalk or paved off-road paths.
* Stay away from any other vehicles.
* Keep your scooter on smooth surfaces and away from sand, dirt, gravel, and water.

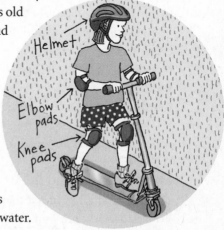

Helmet

Elbow pads

Knee pads

* Always be sure to wear shoes with closed toes and laces tied tight while riding a scooter.
* Avoid bumps and look for possible objects in your path.
* Always face the scooter's handlebars while riding. Do not ride sideways.
* Keep a watchful eye for pedestrians, and cars pulling out of or into driveways, or cars backing up.
* Get off of the scooter and walk it across any crosswalks.

Bike helmets are not for skateboarding. Helmets are designed to protect the head from the impact most likely to occur in a specific sport or set of very similar sports. If you have a bicycle helmet that meets CPSC standards, it will have a label indicating this and that it can also be worn while roller skating, in-line skating, and riding a nonpowered scooter or a low-speed motor-assisted scooter. Helmets for skateboarding must meet a different standard; a label should state that it meets either ASTM F1492 or Snell N-94 requirements.

Be sure your child is ready for in-line skates. Most kids can acquire the skills required for in-line skating when they're around 7 or 8 years old, according to the American Academy of Pediatrics. However, the AAP notes that readiness for in-line skating depends on a combination of factors. Some of these factors are physical, including foot size, body strength, general athletic ability and large-muscle coordination. Other factors are behavioral, including the ability to look out for surface debris and defects and attentiveness to traffic. So readiness for in-line skating is really a judgment call that parents or guardians need to make. If your child is clamoring for in-line skates before you think he is ready, consider starting him with traditional four-wheel skates, which might be easier to control.

In-line skates should fit properly. Your child won't be able to control her in-line skates if they are too big. Make sure there is no room behind the heel once your child slides her foot inside.

The Safe Way to Cross the Street

A child doesn't know that a driver might not see her even if she sees him. She also can't judge the speed a car is going, and she doesn't know that it takes time for a vehicle to stop, particularly in rain and snow. Teach her to wait for a vehicle to come to a complete stop and make eye contact with the driver before entering a crosswalk. Here are other important habits to instill:

• Cross only with an adult or older friend.
• Cross only at an intersection that has traffic signals.
• Use the crosswalk.
• Watch for turning vehicles, and wait for them to turn before crossing.
• Stop at the curb. Look left, right, left, and over your shoulder for traffic. Continue to look as you cross the street.
• Stop to look around parked cars or other objects that block the view of traffic. Let oncoming traffic pass, then look again before crossing. Look both ways as you cross.

Teach safe skating. Your child should always wear a helmet certified for skating, not a bike helmet, as well as knee pads and elbow pads. Supervise your child until she has the skills to skate alone. Beginners should skate in a controlled environment, such as a roller rink or a smooth, paved playground area until they learn how to brake, slow down and turn. Even when she becomes proficient your child should skate on smooth, flat surfaces, including sidewalks and paved trails. She should avoid areas with traffic, making sure to obey the rules of the road when she does enter a crosswalk or road.

Safety rules for pedestrians. While every kid is different, most don't have the judgment to cope with traffic by themselves until they are around 10 years old. But even kindergartners can begin to understand safety rules for pedestrians. Remember, children will learn by your example. Go over the safety rules whenever you have the opportunity, and practice them. Hold your child's hand while crossing the street until he understands and can execute basic pedestrian safety.

Don't run into the street. No matter how many times you have told your child, tell her again—never run out into the street. Don't run after a ball or toy, and don't dart out between parked cars. She might not realize that a neighbor is backing out of a driveway or that someone is quickly turning the corner.

Look for a safe place to walk. Look for streets with sidewalks and wide shoulders. Avoid streets with overgrown bushes, dangerous ditches, trash bins, or parked cars. Try to find streets with crosswalks and traffic signals so your child can cross easily and safely. Look for crossing guards near schools to help children.

Be aware of the bus danger zone. This is the area on all sides of the bus where children are in the most danger of being hit. Your child should stay as far away from the bus as possible unless he is boarding or exiting. At a minimum he should stay 10 feet away from the front and sides of the bus and should never walk behind it. Teach your kids to take five giant steps out from the front of the bus and then wait for the driver to signal that it's OK to cross.

Move away from the bus carefully after exiting. Even though drivers are not supposed to pass a bus as children are leaving it, some still do. Your child needs to make sure that no cars are passing the bus before she moves away from it. After the bus driver signals that it's OK to cross in front, your child should then look to her left and right to make sure no cars are passing before she crosses the street.

Tell your child to take his time getting on or off the bus. He should never hurry. You don't want him to trip and fall under, behind, or in front of the bus. And he should wait for the driver to signal that it's OK to board. Children should board the bus one at a time.

Horseplay should not be allowed around the bus stop. It takes only a moment for a child to fall in front of or under a bus.

Never pick up something near a bus. Tell your child that no matter how important the item is, she should never bend down to pick it up. The driver can't see her, and she could be hit by the bus or slip under it. If she drops something, she should tell the driver and let him or the bus monitor retrieve it.

No dangling straps or drawstrings. Long straps from backpacks or clothing can get caught in the bus door or on the handrail. Make sure your child's clothing and gear are free of anything dangling—key chains, drawstrings at the neck or waist, scarves, belts with tassels, necklaces, purse straps, backpack straps or other items. Loose or long items of clothing should be avoided too. Make your child aware of these hazards.

Is your bus stop in a dangerous location? Talk to your school about changing the location of the bus stop if you have any concerns about its safety.

CHAPTER 13

The Playground

Whether they are at parks, schools or day-care centers, we expect playgrounds to be safe havens for our children. Unfortunately, they are often fraught with hazards. According to the Consumer Products Safety Commission (CPSC), an estimated 200,000 children are treated in emergency rooms every year for injuries related to playground equipment.

You can attack the problem of playground safety on two fronts: First, you can avoid accidents by making sure your child knows how to use the equipment safely, and uses only age-appropriate items; and second, you can keep an eye out for unsafe equipment and conditions. If you find a problem, report it to your parks department, or the principal or a teacher at your school or day-care center.

Dress your child appropriately. Think about your child's clothing and accessories before you head to the playground, and pay attention to both when you're there. She shouldn't wear necklaces, rings, bracelets, backpacks, scarves, or anything else that could get caught. Be sure her clothing doesn't have drawstrings, which can pose a strangulation or injury hazard if they catch on the equipment. If you find a drawstring on children's clothing, report it to the Consumer Product Safety Commission (CPSC) at 800-638-2772 or at *www.cpsc.gov*. Never let your child wear her bicycle helmet on playground equipment; the strap is a strangulation hazard. The helmet can also become wedged in openings in playground equipment, trapping your child's head.

Avoid congested playgrounds. A well-designed playground will be organized into different areas to prevent injuries caused by conflicting activities and kids running between activities. Popular, heavy-use equipment should be spread out to prevent crowding on any one area. Play equipment, open fields, and sand boxes should be located in different sections. Moving equipment such as swings and merry-go-rounds should be off to the side or in a corner with enough space around it to keep kids from running into each other. Teach your child to watch out for children running wildly or children with little parental supervision. Also be aware of overloaded play equipment. Remove your child from crowded climbing equipment, for example, so he doesn't get hurt.

Is the playground surrounded by fencing? There should be fencing between the playground and the parking lot or the street to prohibit little ones from running into a dangerous situation. Your child should not have access to the parking lot or road. Fences and walls should be located at least 6 feet from a swing structure.

Watch out for water hazards. Is there a pond or fountain at your park or playground? Is it accessible to your child? Keep him away from all possible water hazards. Teach him to stay away from the water's edge.

Keep your eyes and at least one hand on him if you decide to feed the ducks or fish.

Make sure playground equipment is placed over appropriate surfacing. It should never be placed over grass, asphalt, concrete, or packed dirt. Falling on grass is as likely to cause injury as a fall onto concrete. The playground should have 12-inch-deep loose fill— engineered wood fiber, wood chips, wood mulch, pea gravel, sand, shredded rubber, or rubber tiles—for equipment up to 6 feet in height. If your playground doesn't have proper surfacing around the equipment, call your local parks department or contact your town to make sure they fix the problem.

How well is your playground equipment maintained? Check the equipment carefully. Look for missing hardware, rusted chains, and rusted or opening S-hooks. Don't put your child on equipment with any of these problems. Warn others about the hazards and contact your town, parks department, or school principal to remedy the situation.

Check the nuts and bolts. Make sure they're not rusted. Rusted nuts and bolts could give way without warning. In addition, look for protruding nuts and bolts that can catch on your child's clothing or cause scrapes or cuts.

Check the ground and the play equipment for protrusions. Swing sets have anchors that should be buried so your child can't fall or trip over them. Check the play area to be sure there aren't anchors, tree roots, rocks, or other obstacles on the ground.

Beware of splinters. Your child should always use play equipment handrails, but keep an eye out for splintering wood. If the playground has wooden playground equipment, see "Take precautions with play sets made of treated wood," page 82.

Watch out for possible pinch-points and sharp edges. Little fingers can fit in places you can't imagine. Watch your child as he explores playground equipment. What may seem benign one moment may lead to a finger entrapment, scrape, or cut in another. If you find one of these hazards, report it to your parks department or school official immediately.

Avoid peeling and chipped paint. Older playground equipment may have been painted with lead-based paint. Stay away from chipped or peeling paint, and be sure your child always washes her hands after playing on any painted equipment. If you're picnicking at the playground, be sure she washes her hands before her meal no matter what equipment she has played on. Playgrounds are notoriously germy.

Look for hazardous debris in the grass or play area. Sometimes our playgrounds and parks don't receive the respect they deserve. Picnickers or fellow playmates might leave behind items that can harm little ones if they step or fall on them, such as broken glass, cans, metal pieces, and bottle caps. Teach your child to watch out for them.

Teach your children to leave debris on the ground. Your child may be fascinated by the trinkets he finds in the grass, loose fill, or sandbox, but he should leave anything he sees where it is. It takes only a split second for him to pick something up and put it in his mouth, hide it in his hand, or store it in his pocket for later.

Be on the lookout for electrical hazards. Watch for exposed electrical wires or boxes in the playground. Tell your child to stay away from these hazards. Report them to your town if you see them.

Supervision is the most important safety measure. Many playground accidents happen due to lack of adult supervision. Don't watch your child from a distance. Stand close to the play equipment he is using and be ready to help if needed. Find out how many adults are supervising your child at his school or childcare facility. Each state has its own staff-to-child ratio for childcare facilities. You can search for the required staff-to-child ratio for child care for all 50 states and the District of Columbia at *nrc.uchsc.edu/STATES/states.htm*, the Web site of the National Resource Center for Health and Safety in Childcare and Early Education.

Make sure equipment is age-appropriate. Your 3-year-old shouldn't play on equipment designed for a 6-year-old. Using equipment meant for a different age group can be deadly. Hanging rings, for example, can be dangerous to small children whose heads may fit through the ring. Signs posted on the playground should clearly indicate the age range for all of the playground equipment. Swings, slides, and climbing equipment are made for preschool-aged children (ages 2 to 5) or for school-aged kids (ages 5 to 12). Even without the signs, you should be able to judge age-appropriateness by the design and scale of the equipment. If you are at all concerned that a piece of equipment may be too high or too difficult for your child, steer clear of it.

Ban monkey bars. If your playground has monkey bars, also called jungle gyms, they should be removed immediately. You might have loved them as a child, but they have proved to be very dangerous. The CPSC estimates that there were 72,000 injuries to children under 10 in 2006 from monkey bars and other climbing equipment. If you see monkey bars on your playground, contact your local parks department to have them removed.

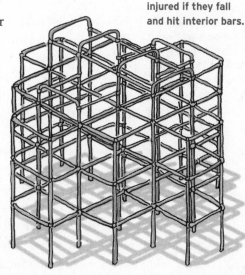

Monkey bars should be removed from playgrounds. Children can be seriously injured if they fall and hit interior bars.

Don't put your child on swing seats made of metal or wood. These harder materials can cause injuries if a child walks in front and gets hit by the swing. The seat should be made of lightweight rubber or plastic. The edges of seats should have smoothly finished or rounded edges, with no protrusions.

Choose a swing that supports your child. If your child is less than 4 years old, he should be placed in a full-bucket tot swing seat that provides protection on all sides of his body. Tot swings should be suspended in their own support structure or at least from a separate bay of the same structure.

Teach your child to walk a safe distance around swings. An accident can easily happen if a child walks too close to a moving swing. She can get hit as the swing moves forward or back or if a kid jumps from a swing. She should walk several feet in front, behind, and to the sides of the swings. If another child is on a swing she wants to use, she should wait until the swing comes to a complete stop before approaching it.

Make sure that your playground has only two swings per bay or structure. Older playgrounds might have three or four swings per bay or structure. This is dangerous because children running behind or in front of the swing set can get struck—and more swings equals greater congestion. Be sure there are only two swings per bay in your playground, and at least 24 inches between the swings, with at least 30 inches between each swing and the side of the bay. Swings should be suspended from support structures that discourage climbing, meaning no horizontal cross bars on A-frames. Only one tire swing is allowed per bay or structure.

Don't let your child play on or near heavy animal swings. These heavy molded plastic and metal animal swings were recalled in 1995 because children can be injured if hit by one. If you see these swings, ask that they be removed immediately.

Heavy plastic and metal swings in the shape of animals can cause injury if they hit a child.

Avoid rope swings. They can fray and wear over time, or they can form a loop that might present a strangulation hazard.

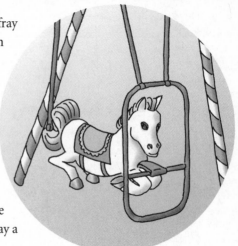

Use tire swings with caution. Supervise your child especially closely while he is on a tire swing. It is often hard to dismount or stop a moving tire swing, especially when used by more than one child. Be sure your child knows to stay a

Tips for Swing Safety

Here are some essential rules to drill into your kids before they get on a swing:

- Hold on with both hands.
- Sit in the center of the swing.
- Never stand or kneel on a swing.
- Don't swing on your stomach.
- Don't play with the chains; they can pinch fingers.
- Stop the swing before getting off.
- Tell the person pushing when you want to get off the swing.
- Don't push other children in the swing.
- Let only adults push you.
- Only one child is allowed on a swing at a time.
- Don't play with the swing when someone else is on it or when it is empty.

safe distance away from all sides of a tire swing when it is in motion. He should not try to climb on or off the tire swing until it has stopped moving. Check to make sure the suspension cable is short enough to prevent kids from swinging into the side supports of the swing frame.

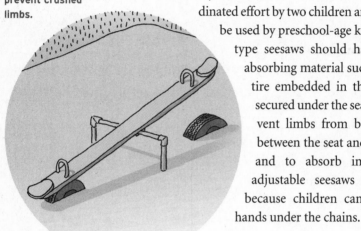

Fulcrum seesaws should have partially buried tires or other shock absorbers to prevent crushed limbs.

Fulcrum seesaws should have shock absorbers. The most familiar type of seesaw (also called a teeter-totter) consists of a board or bar supported in the middle by a fulcrum. These seesaws require a coordinated effort by two children and should not be used by preschool-age kids. Fulcrum-type seesaws should have a shock-absorbing material such as a partial tire embedded in the ground or secured under the seat to help prevent limbs from being crushed between the seat and the ground, and to absorb impact. Avoid adjustable seesaws with chains because children can crush their hands under the chains.

Quick Tips for Safe Climbing

Make sure your kids know these rules before using any climbing equipment:
• Use both hands as well as the correct grip.
• Watch out for other children while climbing.
• Be just as cautious climbing down as climbing up.

• Stay a safe distance away from the child in front of you.
• Climb in the same direction as other children, starting at the same end of the equipment.
• Take your time and climb carefully.
• Don't use climbing apparatus when it's wet.
• Watch out for swinging feet.

Little kids should use spring-centered seesaws. These see-saws use a spring to prevent one side of the seesaw from slamming down if the kid on the other side decides to get off. This is the safest type of see-saw for kids of any age, and the only type that preschool-aged kids should use.

Be sure elevated platforms have proper guardrails or barriers. Equipment designed for preschool-aged children that has a platform higher than 20 inches but less than 30 inches should have a guardrail or protective barrier. (The difference is that a protective barrier is designed to prevent a kid from going through or over it.) If the platform is higher than 30 inches it must have a protective barrier.

Equipment designed for school-age children should have a guardrail or barrier if it is more than 30 inches high. A protective barrier is required if the platform is 48 inches or higher. Equipment may be exempt from this requirement if the guardrail or barrier would interfere with the intended use of the equipment or if it has layered platforms that would prevent a child from falling more than 20 inches.

The slide should fit the child. Some slides are meant for older and physically advanced children. Preschool-aged children should only use slides that are straight or they may use spiral slides if they have only one

The Playground

Quick Tips for Safe Sliding

Here are the rules your kids should know before using a slide:
- Hold onto the ladder with both hands as you climb up the steps of the slide.
- Never climb two steps at a time.
- Don't climb up the front of the slide.
- Slide down sitting up with your feet first.
- Never slide head first.
- No sliding on your stomach.
- No kneeling to slide.
- Only one child should slide down at a time.

turn of 360 degrees or less. A child in this age group has limited ability to maintain balance and postural control.

Check the platform and exit. The platform on any freestanding slide should be at least 22 inches long so kids can comfortably switch from a standing to a sitting position. Platforms should also have a horizontal exit region of at least 11 inches so kids can make a smooth transition from sitting to standing when exiting.

Make sure the bottom of the slide is clear. Teach your child to wait for the child in front of her to move completely off the slide before taking her turn. In addition, she should exit the slide after taking her turn, rather than playing at the bottom. The next child in line might not have her patience.

Is the equipment too hot? Check any metal equipment, such as a slide, before letting your child play on it. A child can easily get a burn from equipment that has been sitting in direct—or even indirect—sunlight.

Don't allow ropes on playground equipment. Your child might like to jump rope at the playground, but she should never take her rope on any equipment. Even if she just holds the rope, it can create a hazard.

Monitor overhead rings and horizontal ladders. These devices are designed for kids at least 4 years old; they require upper body strength and coordination that even a 4- or 5-year-old might not have.

Look for a balance beam that isn't too high. A preschool-aged child shouldn't use a balance beam higher than 12 inches, and a school-aged child shouldn't use one higher than 16 inches.

Supervise merry-go-round use. Don't let your child try to climb on or off a merry-go-round while it's in motion. Preschool-age children should be constantly supervised while on merry-go-rounds. Be sure the the ride has easy-to-use handgrips and that your child knows to hold on tightly and to stay in place once it starts moving.

Don't turn trees into jungle gyms. Your child should learn that trees are meant to be used for shade, not for play. The trees on your local playground (as well as in your yard) should be well-maintained. Dead branches should be cut and dead trees removed to prevent them from falling on anyone. The first 7 feet of tree limbs and branches should be removed so your little ones don't try to climb trees or hang from limbs.

What's in the sandbox? Keep an eye on your child while she's playing in the sandbox and take her out if she finds something dirty or dangerous. Keep her out if the sandbox looks like it hasn't been maintained or cleaned. Ask your parks department to replace the sand regularly. And make sure the sandbox is covered at night.

No standing on the roof! Some playgrounds have houses for children to play in and explore. Tell your child he is not allowed to climb on top of the house. If he falls he could hurt himself and any children below. He shouldn't play in or near the house if others are climbing on the roof— they could fall and hurt him.

Ride on a path. Your child should ride his bicycle only on paths, never in a parking lot and never around playground equipment. If your child rides too close to equipment, there's an increased risk that he'll run into another child or get hit by a swing. Be sure he always wears a helmet and elbow pads when riding. (See "Get in the helmet habit," page 130.)

Keep shoes on. No matter what kind of surfacing is under the play equipment, your child's shoes should remain on her feet at all times. Not only is she in danger from sharp objects, she can also burn her feet if the surfacing is too hot.

CHAPTER 14

Pool and Beach Safety

A trip to the beach or pool is always fun for everyone, and in mid-August it may feel like a welcome relief. But between sand castles and kickboards you need to remember that hazards can accompany water play. Drowning is the second-leading cause of accidental deaths of children ages 1 to 14, according to the Centers for Disease Control's most recent report in 2005.

Drowning can occur when a child leaves the house unnoticed and slips into a pool, or when an adult at poolside momentarily loses sight of him. A child can drown quickly and quietly. Even if your child knows how to swim, he still needs to be monitored constantly. Keep the tips in this chapter in mind so you can enjoy peace of mind as you head to the pool, river, ocean or lake.

Teach your child to swim. You should teach your child to swim when he or she is ready—usually by age five. Of course, knowing how to swim doesn't make children drownproof. An adult should always be present when a child is near water and water safety rules always apply.

Always watch your child near or in water. Whether you are at the beach, a public or private pool, or live near a water hazard such as a well, pond, or stream, you should be at your child's side at all times. Even when there are two caregivers, never take for granted that one is watching your child. According to the Centers for Disease Control (CDC) most young children who drowned in pools were last seen in the house, had been out of sight less than 5 minutes, and were in the care of one or both parents at the time. Typically what happened was the child briefly eluded adult supervision and scampered outside. That's why it is so important to enclose your pool, use a pool alarm, and follow the pool and beach safety tips that come later in this chapter. Also, your child needs to know from the very beginning that he should never swim without adult supervision.

When your children learn to swim, explain the dangers of a rip current and teach them not to try to fight it. Instead they should swim in a direction following the shoreline until they are out of the current, and then they can safely swim to shore.

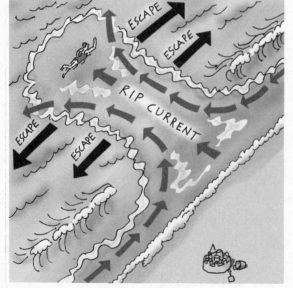

Beware of rip currents. Also known by the misnomer riptides, these currents don't pull you under the water as some people think. They actually carry you out so far you can't get back. They can occur at any beach with waves, even the Great Lakes. You won't be able to see or identify rip currents yourself, so before you leave for the beach, check the latest National Weather Service forecast for local conditions. Many offices also issue a surf zone forecast. Look for posted signs and warning flags at the beach. Check with lifeguards and do exactly what they say. Finally, if in doubt don't go in the water, not even to wade.

Be aware of tide changes. Low tide can change to high tide in a matter of minutes, quickly swamping a beach with water that can be dangerously high if your little one is playing there. Never allow your children to play in sea caves, which may flood with high tide. Refer to tide charts or ask a lifeguard or someone at your hotel so you will know when to expect tide changes.

Select a safe area to swim. If you are swimming in a lake or river, find an area that has good water quality and safe, natural conditions. Avoid murky water, plant life, strong currents, and unexpected drop-offs. Teach children never to swim under any docks, and be sure the docks you use are in good condition—no loose boards or nails. If you are swimming in a bay, river, lake, or ocean, avoid those with big waves and strong tides and currents. Always check local conditions with your hotel or, if renting a house in a beach community, with the local authorities.

Choose a supervised swim area. If you have a choice, a beach, pool, or lake that is watched by trained lifeguards is the safest bet. Even if trained lifeguards are present, you still need to remain vigilant and at your child's side.

Always use a life jacket when boating, fishing, or just sitting on a dock or jetty. A life jacket can be used to help a weak swimmer as well, but your child should only use one that is labeled as U.S. Coast Guard approved. Also check the label on the life jacket to be sure it is intended for your child's weight. Never allow your child in a boat without a life jacket. This same rule applies if he is fishing in a pond or stream.

Stay vigilant around any pool, even a baby pool. You may have purchased a kiddy pool because it appears safer than a large pool, but even a small amount of water requires your constant supervision. (Children can drown in a few inches of water.) You must exercise the same precautions as you would with a tub, and keep your child within arm's reach. Don't put your child in a kiddy pool until he is at least 1 year old.

Empty your child's pool after each use and store it upside down. Not only is your goal to remove the existing water, you also want to turn it upside down so it can't fill with rainwater. Your little one is used to playing in the pool, and if she sees it filled with water—even rain-water—you are inviting trouble.

Choose a hard-sided pool rather than an inflatable pool. It's best to look for a hard-sided pool, but the fact is, most kiddy pools are inflatable, and if you have one of these, you must closely supervise children while in the pool. Always empty the pool and turn it upside down when they are not in it. Once your child is big enough for a larger pool, choose one with hard sides and rigid supports, rather than a larger inflatable pool. Because the sides of an inflatable pool are pliable, it's easier for a child to topple in if she leans on it. However, even hard sides with rigid supports can collapse if a child leans on them, allowing her to slip in, so never leave your child unattended and keep your eyes on him at all times.

Filter pumps for inflatable pools can be dangerous. Some inflatable pools come with portable filter pumps. These pumps do not have ground fault circuit interrupter (GFCI) protection to prevent electrical shock, and because they are not permanently mounted, it is possible for them to wind up in the pool while operating. Additionally, these pumps might not circulate the water frequently enough to keep it clean, and they can be used as climbing platforms by young children.

Many building codes require filter pumps to be permanently connected to in-ground pools. If you have an aboveground pool, use a filter pump that is designed to be permanently mounted. If the pump has a plug instead of being permanently wired, make sure you plug it into a GFCI-protected circuit.

Not all pool covers are safety covers. Safety covers must be made of strong material and must be securely anchored into a concrete or wooden deck. This means they can only be installed over in-ground pools or on aboveground pools that are surrounded by a wooden deck. Do not use clip-on covers for aboveground pools. If a child falls into a pool with a clip-on cover he could get trapped under the cover or entangled in the cover.

The dimensions shown here are intended to make sure a child can't get over, under or through a fence surrounding a pool.

Enclose your pool. If you install an aboveground pool, an in-ground pool, spa or a hot tub, you might be required by state or local regulations to enclose it so that children cannot get unsupervised access. Whether or not law requires enclosure, it's essential for safety. Enclose your pool with non-climbable fencing that is at least 4 feet high and includes a self-closing, self-latching, lockable gate. The latch must be out of the reach of children. The gate should open out from the pool so a child can't open it by pushing on it. If you have a spa or hot tub, at the very

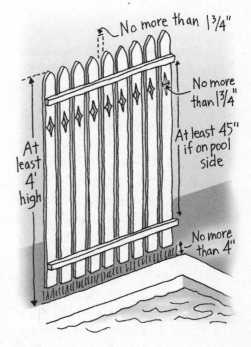

No more than 1¾"

No more than 1¾"

At least 45" if on pool side

At least 4' high

No more than 4"

least make sure it has a cover that securely locks. Be diligent about locking the cover whenever you are not in the spa or hot tub.

- **Be ready for emergencies.** No matter what type of pool your child is using, keep a phone and first-aid kit close by in case of emergency. Learn CPR and always have a life preserver and shepherd's hook in the pool area to pull a child to safety, if necessary.

Remove toys from the water immediately after use. Toys are enticing to a child. You don't want him to try to fish out his favorite ball or reach for the swim float.

Remove toys from the entire pool area. Toys and floats near a pool can be dangerous attractions. If your child sees them she may want to put them in the pool or may inadvertently drop them into the water—and she may want to retrieve them.

Teach your child to ask before jumping or diving. Your child doesn't know the risks of jumping or diving into a pool or other body of water. The only time she should be allowed to jump or dive in is when an adult present knows the depth, knows it is safe, and is sure there aren't any underwater objects that could harm her.

Stow the ladder. If you have an aboveground pool, make sure to secure, lock, or remove the ladder after each use. You can also add fencing that is at least 4 feet high that surrounds the pool, preventing access to the ladder. This way you can control access to the pool while you are in it.

Make sure your pool is equipped with an SVRS. The suction from a water circulation drain can cause a child to become trapped underwater. To prevent this, be sure the drain or drains on your pool have a Safety Vacuum Release System (SVRS) to combat possible suction entrapment. An SVRS will detect strong suction—from a body entrapment, for example—and shut off the pump immediately. You should see this fixture at the filter pump. If you don't have an SVRS, you can get one retrofitted. Some spas and hot tubs also incorporate SVRSs into the design of their circulation system.

Keep kids away from pool drains. Teach your children to stay away from all pool and spa drains, whether or not there are SVRSs. Many incidents involve girls with long, fine hair that gets pulled into a drain. If your child has long hair, make sure she wears a bathing cap or has her hair gathered in a ponytail or bun. Even wading pool drains can be very dangerous; young children have suffered serious internal injuries by sitting on them.

Use safety covers on your pool, spa, or hot tub drains. Anti-entrapment/anti-entanglement covers are designed to keep your child's hair from getting tangled in the drain, thus trapping her. Again, whether or not the drain is fitted with an SVRS, it still needs a safety cover. Proper covers will be dome-shaped or raised, not flat. If your drains don't have proper covers, you can buy them online or at your local pool supply company. Make sure the cover will work with your pool, hot tub or spa. Some will work only on the bottom of a pool, not on a sidewall. Check the drains on hotel pools or any other pool your child uses. If the drains are flat or uncovered, don't let your children use the pool.

Pools, hot tubs, and spas should have raised drain covers to prevent your child from becoming entrapped.

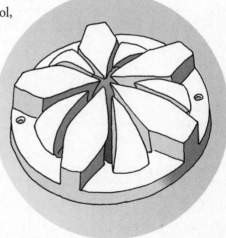

Ban loose jewelry. Necklaces and other loose jewelry can catch in pool drains.

Know where the electrical cut-off switch for the pool or spa pump is located. Be sure that it is clearly marked and that anyone watching children at the pool knows where it is. Shut off the pump immediately if someone is trapped against a drain, bring him to the surface, and call 911 right away.

Install door alarms. Equip all doors that allow access to your swimming pool with an audible alarm. The alarm should be loud and sound for 30 seconds or more within 7 seconds of a door opening. Be sure your door alarm is distinct from any other sound in the house and resets automatically. Adults will want to pass through these doors without setting off the alarm, so install a switch or keypad that will deactivate the alarm for no more than 15 seconds. To keep it out of the reach of children, position this switch or keypad 54 inches above the threshold of the door covered by the alarm. For more protection you can add alarms to your windows as well. They should also make a distinct sound if opened.

Add a pool alarm. There are four types of pool alarms: surface or floating alarms, underwater alarms that detect waves under the surface,

What to Do if Your Child Is Sunburned

Red and painful skin are the most common symptoms of sunburn. If your baby is younger than a year and suffers even mild sunburn, call your doctor immediately; a severe sunburn is considered an emergency at this age. Contact a doctor if a child older than a year gets a sunburn that is severe or forms blisters. You should also seek medical attention if your child has a fever, chills, swelling, nausea, or is vomiting or feeling faint after sun exposure. Don't re-expose your child to the sun until the sunburn has completely healed.

You can use a moisturizing lotion on burned skin but don't rub it in, and do not use salve, butter or ointment on sunburn, or break blisters. If touching the skin is painful, don't apply anything. Use a cold compress, or submerge the burned area in cold water. You can also use calamine lotion but not one with an added antihistamine. You may be able to give an older child acetaminophen for fever and pain, but check with your doctor first. Give your child plenty of liquids, since sunburn can cause dehydration.

pool perimeter alarms, and personal alarms, worn on a wristband that sounds an alarm when exposed to water. Look for an alarm that meets the ASTM standards and has a remote alarm receiver so that it can be heard inside the house or in other areas away from the pool. The standard for these alarms is voluntary; as a result, not all pool alarms are reliable, and they are not a substitute for fencing, door alarms, and adult supervision. They are just an added measure of security. Keep in mind that a personal alarm works only if the child doesn't figure out how to remove it, and of course, it doesn't protect neighborhood kids who are not wearing one.

Electrical devices are a no-no. Keep electrical devices such as TVs, radios, and CD players out of the pool area.

A flotation device is not necessarily a safety device. In fact, some flotation devices can give you and your child a false sense of security. Your child should only wear a life vest that has been approved by the U.S. Coast Guard. Inflatable devices such as rafts and toys can lose air, shift positions, or slip out from underneath your child. Remember, too, that no flotation device is a substitute for your close supervision. Don't let a child who cannot swim use an inflatable toy or mattress in water that is above the waist.

Have your pool or spa regularly inspected. Be sure to hire an experienced pool technician to check for hazards that could lead to entrapment or entanglement, and to check the working condition of any pumps, drains, and SVRS. Ask for an inspection of the drain suction fittings and covers on your pool and spa; you need to be sure they are properly attached and are the proper size. Ask if they meet current safety standards.

Look in the pool first. If your child is missing, every second counts. Be sure to look in the pool first. Go to the edge of the pool and examine the entire pool—the bottom and the surface, as well as the surrounding area.

Secure umbrellas. If you are using a beach or pool umbrella or a beach tent, be sure the poles are secure. If the wind picks them up someone could be injured by a flying umbrella or tent peg.

Keep babies out of the sun. A new baby's skin burns more easily, so try to avoid any sun exposure, especially direct exposure, until he is 6 months old. Keep his skin covered, even in the shade. You shouldn't routinely use sunscreen on a baby less than 1 year old, but it's OK to use if you find yourself in a situation where you can't keep him out of the sun. Use a broad-spectrum sunscreen that's made specifically for children with an SPF of at least 15. If your baby is less than 6 months old, apply the sunscreen to a small area of his back first to make sure there is no irritation, and then apply only to face and hands. And keep the rest of him covered up.

After 1 year, break out the sunscreen. Young children should stay out of the sun as much as possible, but of course that gets harder to accomplish as they get older and more active and independent. When you child reaches 1 year, you can apply sunscreen regularly. Apply it 30 minutes before she goes outside and reapply it every two hours—more often if she goes swimming or is sweating. Be careful not to get sunscreen on the eyelids. As with babies, use a waterproof, broad-spectrum sunscreen made for children with a SPF of at least 15.

Cover up to protect skin at any age. A hat with a 3-inch brim or a bill facing forward and a long-sleeved shirt and long pants made from tightly woven cotton provide smart protection against the sun. Keep in mind that sand and concrete reflect the sun's rays, increasing the chances of a burn. Most rays make it through a cloud cover and they also travel through water, so an overcast day or staying in the pool doesn't provide protection.

CHAPTER 15

Stings, Bites, Burns, and Poisoning

A sting is painful for an adult; imagine how it feels to a child who is stung for the first time. He's in for a real shock if he's stung by a bee or a wasp such as a hornet or yellow jacket. Bites, burns, and poisoning, along with stings, are scary for both you and your child. The last thing you want is to be frantically trying to figure out what to do while your child is screaming in pain. This chapter will arm you with the information you need so you can act quickly, effectively, and calmly as you soothe your child and work to ease his pain.

Avoid attracting bees or wasps. Wear light-colored clothing and steer clear of perfumes and scented soaps to avoid stings. If you are picnicking, put food away when you've finished; don't leave food and drinks uncovered. Also be sure to put your garbage in a covered can. Picnic in a shaded area away from flowering plants, not in an open area. And remember, bees are most active when the weather is warm.

Don't swing or swat. This might rile the insect and cause it to sting. Tell your child to remain still if a stinging insect is nearby. If a bee or other stinging insect stings your child, bring her inside immediately—if one bee stings, others often follow.

Remove the stinger immediately—and carefully. If your child is stung by a bee or wasp, try scraping the stinger away by grazing it with a credit card, a blunt-edged object, or, if nothing else is handy, a fingernail in a side-to-side motion. Avoid using tweezers; squeezing the stinger or pulling it might push more venom into the skin. Removing the stinger right away can reduce the severity of the sting because it takes the stinger a few minutes to pump all its venom into the victim.

Relieve the pain from a sting. After removing the stinger, wash the affected area with soap and water. You may be able to relieve some of the pain with a compress of ice wrapped in a cloth so it won't freeze the skin. Keep the compress on for 10 minutes and then off for 10 minutes. Talk to your doctor about over-the-counter pain creams and oral medications.

A credit card is one effective tool you might have on hand to scrape a bee stinger out of your child's skin.

Watch for allergic reactions to stings. Check your child for hives, dizziness, difficulty breathing, tightness in his chest or throat, nausea or vomiting, persistent pain, or swelling. If he is experiencing any of those symptoms, call 911 immediately. Parents who are allergic should keep a very close eye on their children for similar reactions.

Prepare for stings if your child is allergic to them. Your doctor might recommend that you carry epinephrine, a prescription hormone, if your child has had an allergic reaction to a sting in the past.

Seek immediate help for a mouth or nose sting. If your child is stung in the mouth or nose, the resulting swelling could inhibit his breathing. Call for medical attention immediately.

Scratching can cause infection. Your child may want to scratch the area where she has been stung. Don't let her do this because it could irritate the area and increase the risk of infection. To further reduce the risk of infection, wash the area several times each day for the next few days and watch for signs of infection, such as increased redness, swelling, or pain. Because stingers puncture the skin, there is also a risk of tetanus. So check with your doctor to see if your child should have a tetanus booster.

Always keep an eye out for ticks. If you are walking in the woods or by a lake or if you are visiting or live in an area with deer, be on the lookout for ticks. They carry Lyme disease and Rocky Mountain spotted fever. If you are going on a hike, don't let your children touch plants and instruct them to walk in the middle of the trail and stay away from long grasses.

Dress your child in light-colored clothing. Ticks stand out on light-colored clothes. Dress your child in long sleeves and pants, and tuck his pants into his socks so ticks can't get to his skin. A tick may still be able to get into shoes or socks, so be sure to check his feet and ankles (and

What to Do if Your Child Is Burned

How you treat a burn in the first few minutes after it occurs can make a huge difference in the severity of the injury. Remove all burned clothing; however, if clothing adheres to the skin, cut or tear around burned areas. Remove all jewelry, belts, tight clothing, etc. from over the burned areas and from around the victim's neck. This is very important because burned areas swell immediately. Here are the types of burns and their treatment, from the Centers for Disease Control and Prevention.

First-degree burns involve the top layer of skin only. Sunburn is a first-degree burn. (See "What to Do If Your Child Is Sunburned," page 158.) Skin will be red, painful to touch, and will show mild swelling.

Second-degree burns involve the first two layers of skin. Skin will be deep red and painful. It may have a glossy appearance from leaking fluid, and there may be blisters and possible loss of some skin.

Treatment
- Apply cool, wet compresses or immerse in cool fresh water until pain subsides.
- Cover the burn with a sterile, nonadhesive bandage or clean cloth.
- You can use over-the-counter medications to help relieve pain and reduce inflammation, but don't give aspirin to a child or teenager.
- First-degree burns usually heal without further treatment. However, if the burn covers a large area of the body or if the victim is an infant, seek emergency medical attention.

Treatment
- Immerse in fresh, cool water or apply cool compresses. Continue for 10 to 15 minutes.
- Dry with a clean cloth and cover with sterile gauze.
- Do not break blisters.
- Elevate burned arms or legs.
- Take steps to prevent shock: Lay the child flat, elevate his feet about 12 inches, and cover the child with a coat or blanket. However, do not place the victim in this shock position if a head, neck, back, or leg injury is suspected, or if it makes the victim uncomfortable.
- Further medical treatment is required. Do not attempt to treat serious burns unless you are a trained health professional. If a second-degree burn covers an area more than 2 to 3 inches in diameter, or if it is located on the hands, feet, face, groin, buttocks, or a major joint, treat the burn as a major one.

Third-degree burns penetrate the entire thickness of the skin and permanently destroy tissue. They are often painless, although pain may be caused by patches of first- and second-degree burns, which often surround third-degree burns. The skin is dry and leathery and may appear charred or have patches, which appear white, brown or black. There also may be loss of skin layers.

Treatment

- Cover burn lightly with sterile gauze or clean cloth.
- Take steps to prevent shock. Lay the child flat and elevate his feet about 12 inches.
- Have him sit up if his face is burned. Watch closely for possible breathing problems.
- Elevate burned area higher than the child's head when possible. Keep him warm and comfortable. Watch for signs of shock, including pale, clammy skin, weakness, bluish lips and fingernails, and a drop in alertness.
- Do not place a pillow under your child's head if he is lying down and there is an airway burn. (See airway burns, at right.) This can close the airway.
- Immediately call for medical attention. Do not attempt to treat serious burns unless you are a trained health professional.

What not to do

- Don't apply medications, cream, oil spray, ice or any household remedy. Ointments or butter might cause infection.
- Don't breathe, blow, or cough on the burn.
- Don't use bandage material that can leave lint on the burn.
- Don't disturb blistered skin.
- Don't remove clothing that is stuck to the skin.
- Don't give the child anything by mouth if there is a severe burn.
- Don't immerse a severe burn in cold water. This can cause shock.

Airway burns These burns can be very serious since the rapid swelling of burned tissue in the airway can quickly block air flow to the lungs. They can be caused by inhaling smoke, steam, superheated air, or toxic fumes, often in a poorly ventilated space. If there is a chance your child was exposed to any of those causes, immediately call for emergency medical help. Symptoms include burns on the lips; burns on the head, face, or neck; wheezing; a change in voice, difficulty breathing; coughing; singed nose hairs or eyebrows; and dark mucus.

Burn follow-up

Most minor burns heal without further treatment. However, call your doctor if pain persists for more than 48 hours or if signs of infection develop—increased pain, redness, swelling, drainage, red streaks spreading from the burn, or fever.

✳ **Stings, Bites, Burns, and Poisoning**

entire body—see below) when you return from any place that might harbor ticks.

Check your child's entire body for ticks. Look everywhere, even hard-to-reach areas and less obvious places, including in and around her ears, in her hair, on her scalp, inside her belly button, under her arms, on the backs of her knees, her genitals, between her buttocks, and around her waist. Children can't check themselves over, so this is your responsibility.

Check Fido too. Pets can easily carry ticks into the house, so be sure to check them after an outdoor ramble. It's best not to let pets run free in wooded areas; they can expose the family to poison ivy as well as ticks.

Remove any ticks you find. Use fine-tipped tweezers to firmly grasp the tick very close to your child's skin. With a steady motion, pull the tick's body away from the skin; do not twist. Then clean the skin with soap and warm water. Place the dead tick in a sealable plastic bag marked with the date and store it in the freezer. This way the tick can be tested for disease if your child becomes ill.

Look for a bull's-eye rash. A circular rash, often with the appearance of a bull's eye in the center, is often the first sign of Lyme disease. The bull's eye appears as the rash expands and the center of the rash clears. Additional circular rashes may appear as well. Your child may not have this rash (or you may not see it before it disappears), so you must look out for other symptoms, which include a fever, headache, fatigue, chills,

Remove a tick by pulling straight up with tweezers.

muscle and joint aches, and swollen lymph nodes. If you see this rash or your child experiences any of these symptoms, contact her doctor immediately.

Look for Rocky Mountain spotted fever. Although it's named after the region where it was first discovered, Rocky Mountain spotted fever now occurs throughout the United States from April through September. Early symptoms include fever, nausea, vomiting, muscle pain, lack of appetite, and severe headache. Later symptoms include rash, abdominal pain, joint pain, and diarrhea. It can be a severe illness, and the majority of patients are hospitalized.

A bull's-eye rash is one symptom that may occur in some cases of Lyme disease.

Apply repellent carefully. Some insect repellents may react with your child's skin and cause a rash. Repellents can also cause irritation to the eyes and can be potentially fatal if swallowed. If using a repellent on your child, avoid her eyes and mouth. Also avoid putting repellent on her hands because she can transfer it to her eyes or mouth. Don't apply too much. Your child doesn't need to be saturated with it for it to work. You can use a repellent with 10 percent or more deet on skin or clothing, but you should not use a product with a concentration of more than 30 percent for your infant or child. Reapply repellent only as often as recommended on the label.

Do not use deet under clothing, over cuts or wounds, or on irritated skin. The U.S. Environmental Protection Agency (EPA) has found deet to be safe when used according to directions on the label. But be sure to wash your child with soap and water when she returns home. And don't use repellents on infants less than 2 months old.

Look for age restrictions on insect repellents. Oil of lemon eucalyptus, a plant-based repellent, for example, has been found to provide similar protection to low concentrations of deet but should not be used on children under the age of 3. If the repellent has an age restriction, it must be stated on the product. If you don't see one, the EPA has not mandated one.

Keep insect repellents out of reach of your children. When you have finished using a repellent, store it out of your child's reach in a locked cabinet.

Wash clothing after using repellent. If you have sprayed your child with repellent or sprayed it on his clothing, wash the clothes before letting him wear them again.

Use mosquito netting over your infant carrier or stroller. If you are planning to be outside hiking or picnicking, or in an area with biting or stinging insects, protect your child by keeping her covered with long pants and sleeves and by using mosquito netting designed specifically for a stroller or infant carrier. Be sure the netting isn't too long—your child could get tangled in it.

Safeguard against mosquitoes. Infected mosquitoes spread the West Nile virus. The results can be serious or even fatal. Use age-appropriate insect repellent and make sure your child wears long sleeves and long pants if he's venturing into an area potentially filled with mosquitoes. Mosquitoes need standing water to breed. So eliminate places where standing water can collect in your yard, including wheelbarrows, buckets and birdbaths. Be cautious even in cooler weather when you wouldn't expect mosquitoes to be a problem. Mosquitoes are most active at dusk and through the evening, so try to keep your kids inside at that time.

Beware of spider bites

Two types of spiders found in the U.S. are dangerous to humans: the black widow and the brown recluse. The black widow is commonly found outdoors in woodpiles, rubble piles, under stones, in hollow stumps, and in sheds and garages. Inside you might run into them in undisturbed, cluttered areas in basements and crawl spaces. The brown recluse builds small retreat webs behind objects of any type. Teach your child not to disturb a spider web.

• The adult female black widow is about ½-inch long, normally shiny black, with a red or orange hourglass marking on their abdomen. Bitten skin may display a "target" appearance, with a pale area surrounded by a red ring—or the bite may go unnoticed. Pain progresses from the bite site to the abdomen and back, with possible severe cramping, nausea, tremors, profuse perspiration, restlessness, and fever. Wash the wound well with soap and water, then apply ice to slow absorption of venom. If the bite is on an arm or leg, keep it elevated. Seek immediate medical attention. There are medications to treat all the symptoms. Bites are rarely lethal, but your child might be held overnight for observation.

• The brown recluse spider is ¼- to ¾-inch long, golden brown, and has a dark violin-shaped marking on the top. Bite symptoms vary. First symptoms are pain, burning and itching. The bite becomes reddened within several hours and takes on a bull's-eye appearance, with a center blister surrounded by a red ring and then a white ring. There is often a systemic reaction within 24 to 36 hours, with fever, chills, a possible rash, nausea, weakness, and joint pain. Clean the bite with soap and water and apply ice. If the bite is on an arm or leg, keep it elevated. Seek immediate medical attention. Your doctor might use antibiotics to treat infection. Tissue at the bite area will die and be sloughed off as the bite heals.

Relieve the pain of a common spider bite with a cool compress. Be sure to clean the area of the bite with soap and water first. Don't give aspirin to a child or teenager. If your child is in pain, ask your doctor whether he can have acetaminophen.

Brown recluse

Black widow

Bites from these spiders are dangerous and require medical attention.

Teach your child to stay away from unfamiliar animals. Animals that appear friendly or are cute can still bite, scratch, or have rabies, including adorable dogs and cats. Each year, about 400,000 children need medical attention for dog bites. This includes all children, not just infants or toddlers. Almost two-thirds of injuries among children 4 and younger are to the head or neck region. Rabies is a disease of mammals but is much more common among wild animals. Most-common carriers are skunks, raccoons, beavers, squirrels, bats, foxes, and coyotes. But even a cute goat at a petting zoo can transmit it.

Supervise children around pets. You might have a sweet older dog or cat that you would never imagine could ever bite or scratch anyone. But even the most docile pet can be provoked into biting or scratching if a small child decides to pull on the pet's ears or tail, or otherwise inadvertently hurts the animal. So don't let your little ones play with your pets unless you are within arm's reach.

Wash a dog or cat bite or scratch immediately and thoroughly for at least five minutes, then call the doctor. Bites, especially around the head or face, require medical attention. If the animal is a stray, call animal control. If you know the owner, find out if the animal has been vaccinated. If your child needs a rabies shot, it must be given as soon as possible. If you have a pet, keep all vaccinations up to date. If a wild animal bites your pet, your pet could be infected, so call your veterinarian immediately.

Know what the poison ivy plant looks like. It can be found as a low-growing shrub or as a vine that trails along the ground or climbs to the top of a tree. Look for groups of three leaflets along the stem. The leaves, which may or may not appear waxy, are typically greenish-red in the spring and dark green in the summer. They change color in the fall to shades of red, yellow, and orange. The best way to teach your kids how to avoid poison ivy is to drill this old saying into their heads: "Leaves of three, let it be."

Recognize poison ivy symptoms. Exposure to poison ivy will result in red bumps and large, weeping blisters, erupting into streaks or patches where the plant touched the skin, plus extreme itching. If your child came in contact with the poison ivy oil by brushing against a plant, the rash will be linear. If she got it from a piece of clothing the rash will be more dispersed.

Stop the spread of poison ivy. While scratching a poison-ivy rash will cause more damage and possibly infection, it won't spread the rash even if the blisters break. It's the oil on the plant that causes the rash. If your child gets the oil on his hands and touches other parts of his body, those areas can also break out. He can get the rash from clothing that has been contaminated with the oil from poison ivy. He doesn't need to come into direct contact with the actual plant.

A poison-ivy rash might not appear right away. So if you suspect your child has come in contact with poison ivy—or even if you spot poison ivy in a place he may have been playing—he should wash immediately to remove the oil and prevent further spreading. Wash his hands first, using a nailbrush to be sure you clean under his fingernails. A poison-ivy rash usually breaks out within 12 to 48 hours of contact, but it can appear anywhere from 4 hours to 10 days after contact.

"Leaves of three, let it be" is the best way to teach your children to avoid the misery of poison ivy.

Poison-ivy rashes can clear up on their own. While the rashes can often clear up in one to three weeks without treatment, your child might need a topical ointment or prescription to alleviate the pain and discomfort. That's important to help the child resist damaging scratching.

The rash might look like it's spreading. Don't be alarmed if the rash seems to creep along your child's skin. This is due to the time it takes for the skin to react to the oily resin.

If the rash affects your child's eyes or mouth, consult a doctor. In addition, if your child develops a fever, the rash is severe, his blisters ooze, or the rash doesn't clear up within a few weeks, call your child's doctor.

Don't give syrup of Ipecac for poisoning. If your child ingests a poisonous substance or one you suspect is poisonous, do not give him syrup of Ipecac or anything that will make him throw up the poison. Call the poison control center first. The substance he ingested might do more harm coming back up than it did going down.

Proper storage is a key to preventing poisoning. Store household products and medicines in locked cabinets that your child can't reach. Do not store them over stoves or ovens. Keep medicines in child-resistant containers, read labels and double check with your pediatrician before dispensing them to your children. Each medicine should be clearly labeled. And never try to entice your child into taking medicine by referring to it as candy.

Don't transfer products or medicines to other containers. Every household product should be in its original container with the label intact. In the event of a poisoning, you will need to give the poison-control center vital information listed on the container and on the label.

Beware of possible drug interactions. Before giving your child any medicine—whether prescription or over-the-counter—tell your

Know How to Call for Help if Poisoning Occurs

You can reach your local poison center by calling 800-222-1222. Keep this number near all your phones. Someone is available to answer calls 24 hours a day, seven days a week. Be sure your caregiver or anyone watching your child is aware of the number and keeps it on or near their phones as well.

Poison centers answer nonemergency calls as well as emergency calls. For example, you can call for information about poison prevention or to find out about drug interactions, poisonous plants, and safe pesticide use.

doctor about any other medicine she is taking to prevent adverse drug interactions. It is a good idea to check with a pharmacist as well, if you have questions, or if your child is taking more than one over-the-counter drug. Check the label on any medication to see when it should be taken and under what conditions (with or without food or dairy products, for example).

Poisons don't have to be ingested to be dangerous. Many household cleaners are dangerous if ingested, inhaled, or splashed. If poison is splashed, rinse the area with water for 15 minutes. And no matter what type of contact your child has had with those substances, call the poison center immediately.

Poisons come in solid, liquid, or sprayable forms, and some are even invisible. Teach your child that poisons come in all shapes and sizes, and even in bright and appealing colors, like colorful medicine capsules or fruit-tinted cleaning products. A poison can taste, smell, or look good, for example, a mouthwash or perfume. Invisible poisons can be found in something burning, such as fumes from your vehicle exhaust.

Don't breathe vapors. Never sniff containers to determine what's inside. This could lead to poisoning from inhaling. Before you start using

Be Aware of These Household Poisons

The National Capital Poison Center has listed some household items that are dangerous for children. If you use any of these products, buy them in small quantities and keep them away from your children. Discard what you no longer need.

- Alcoholic beverages
- Antifreeze
- Artificial nail-glue remover
- Automatic dishwasher detergents
- Dietary supplements (especially with iron) and herbals/botanicals
- Drain openers
- Furniture polish
- Gasoline,
- Kerosene
- Lamp oil
- Medicines (prescription and over-the-counter)
- Miniature batteries
- Mouthwash
- Oven cleaner
- Paint thinner
- Pesticides
- Toilet-bowl cleaners
- Windshield wiper solution

household and chemical products, turn on fans and open windows to ventilate the room to avoid inhaling dangerous chemicals. If your child breathes in poisonous vapors, get him fresh air and call the poison center.

Don't let children play in pesticide-treated areas. If your lawn has been sprayed with pesticides, keep your children away from it. Pesticides can be absorbed through the skin and can be extremely poisonous. Remove toys before spraying. If a pesticide company sprays for you, it should leave a warning sign on your lawn and tell you when it is safe for children to play on it again. Of course, if you have kids you can always skip the lawn pesticides altogether until they are older.

Learn more about pesticides. Call the National Pesticide Information Center at 800-858-7378. The phones are open from 6:30 a.m. to 4:30 p.m. Pacific Time, 7 days a week. Or you can email the experts at *npic@ace.orst.edu* or visit the Web site at *npic.orst.edu* if you have any questions regarding when you should use pesticides, the different types of pesticides, how they work, and how to use them safely.

CHAPTER 16

Fire Safety

No one wants to think about the possibility of a house fire, but it's something you need to plan for in order to protect your family. Every year about 400,000 residential fires are reported to fire departments, and they kill about 3,000 people a year, according to the U.S. Fire Administration. An escape plan that includes working smoke detectors will increase your chance of escaping a fire. With our busy and hectic lives, it's all too easy to postpone practicing for a fire, but you and your family should create a plan and practice now. The safety tips in this chapter will help to prevent a fire and survive if one does occur.

Know how to use a fire escape ladder. If your home has two or more floors, keep a fire escape ladder in each bedroom. If your child is too little to use it, keep it out of his reach so he won't be tempted to play with it. When your child becomes capable of safely using the ladder on his own, keep it near a window and make sure he knows where

Plan primary and secondary escape routes and one for each person living in your house. Include a spot outside where everyone can meet.

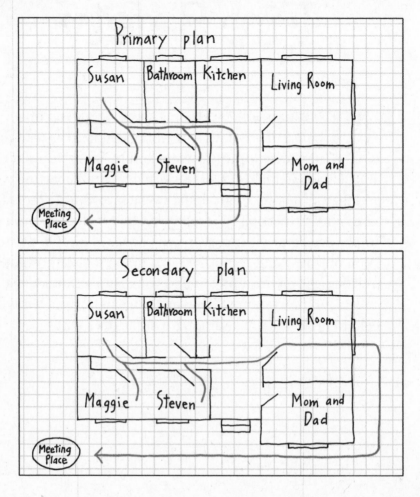

it is and how to use it. Practice setting up the escape ladder and exiting, but only from a first floor window. There must always be an adult present; tell your children never to practice on their own.

Create a fire escape plan. Draw a sketch of your house with at least two routes you and your children can take from each room in order to exit the house in case one of the routes is blocked. The escape routes should include doors and windows; so make sure they can be opened easily. You and your children should practice each route.

Make a plan for each child. If you're a two-parent household with more than one child, decide which adult will get which child, how each of you plans to get out of the house, and where you will meet once you have escaped. Have an alternate strategy in case one parent is not home during a fire. Children around the age of 11 or 12 are usually responsible enough and physically able to get out of the house themselves, although every child is different so you will have to use your judgment. If you do decide to allow a child to escape on his own, make sure he knows exactly what to do. And make sure the other children know to wait for you to come get them. If possible, have a back-up person assigned to pick up a baby or young child, just in case the person assigned isn't home. Update the plan as your kids get older.

You Might Need Voice Alarms

As piercing as the sound of a conventional alarm is, don't be surprised if it doesn't wake up one or more of your kids when you do your nighttime fire drill. A study of 24 children published in Pediatrics, the journal of the American Academy of Pediatrics, found that a conventional alarm woke only 14 of them from a deep sleep. If you have this problem, try a personalized smoke alarm. With these alarms you record a message calling out to your children by name to wake them up, along with simple instructions telling them what to do. This alarm woke 23 children from a deep sleep. Neither alarm woke the 24th child.

Decide how you will carry your baby. Keep on hand a baby harness or baby carrier of some type that will allow you to keep your hands free to help you escape. The harness should be by the crib or bassinet so you are ready in an emergency.

Explain your fire escape plan. Sit down with your family and tell them what you have created. Be sure everyone knows exactly what he or she is supposed to do in the event of a fire. Review the plan with caregivers and older family members as well. Children as young as 3 can follow a fire-escape plan if they understand it and have some practice. Your goal should be to have everyone out of the house in no more than 3 minutes. Remind your children not to stop to take a favorite toy or anything else with them.

Clear all exits. Don't allow doorways, or window areas if they are to be used as exits, to be blocked or obstructed by toys, jackets, shoes, or miscellaneous items. You don't want to have any obstacles on the floor in the event of a fire. If your windows or doors have security bars, make sure that the bars have quick-release devices. Teach your children how to release the bars, making it clear that they are to be opened only in an emergency.

Conduct fire drills at least twice a year. Set off all the alarms in the daytime so your children know what they'll hear in case of a fire. If the drill doesn't work as expected, explain to your children what went wrong—and what went right. Once your kids have mastered your fire-escape plan, do the drill at night.

Sleep with bedroom doors closed. This may prevent smoke from overwhelming you or your child, possibly allowing extra time for firefighters to reach you. But closed doors may prevent you from hearing a smoke alarm that goes off in a child's room, so put a baby monitor in each child's room so you can hear the alarm, and test to be sure that you can distinguish the sound of the smoke alarm as heard through the baby monitor.

Teach your children not to hide from fire or firefighters. If you have young children who are not yet capable of following an escape plan on their own, make sure they know that they should wait near a window for someone to come and get them. If possible, they should signal for help with a blanket, towel or flashlight. Tell them not to be afraid of firefighters, who will be in uniforms and possibly wearing masks and may be carrying heavy equipment. Your children should understand that they should not waste time trying to find you. Assure them that someone will come to get them and that person must know where they'll be. You might want to plan a trip to your local firehouse to familiarize your children with the firefighters and some of their equipment.

Teach your children to stay low. Let your children know that they need to be low to the ground to crawl under the smoke. Show them how to reduce the risk of smoke inhalation by covering their nose and mouth. Tell them the best thing to use is a wet towel, but that a T-shirt, pajama top or other cloth item will do. Whatever they use, tell them to bunch it up to keep it small so it can't catch fire.

Stop, drop, and roll. Teach your children that if they see fire on their body or clothing they should immediately stop in their tracks, drop to the floor, cover their face to protect it from the flames, and roll to extinguish the fire. Practice this drill with them.

Teach children to stay low and cover their faces to avoid smoke inhalation.

Check a door before opening it. A child's first instinct in a fire may be to run and open her door. Teach them not to open the door if there is heat or smoke coming through the cracks. If there's no heat or smoke, they should first touch the door and then the doorknob. If both are cool, they can open the door. If they encounter heat or smoke, tell them to make sure the door is tightly closed, then wait for help.

Choose a safe meeting place. Your escape plan should include a safe meeting place outside the home and away from danger. Make sure your children know exactly where to meet and remind them never to go back inside the house. If a family member is missing, tell the emergency

Fire-Safety Tips for Apartment Dwellers

Because apartment buildings have multiple dwellings, levels, and corridors plus long stairways to the street, procedures for escaping a fire are different than for a house. If your escape routes are blocked, you'll need to wait in your apartment for the fire department. If you do follow an escape route, take your key with you in case your way is blocked and you need to return to your apartment. Here are other tips to follow:

• Know the building's evacuation plan. Posted in a public area so you can review it, the plan will illustrate what to do in the event of a fire. If no plan is posted, speak to your landlord. Be sure your management company holds a fire drill at least once a year and that their building's fire safety systems are checked regularly.
• Practice escape routes with your family. Make a sketch of your apartment and the building, identifying the exits. Highlight all stairways in case one is blocked by fire.

• Never use the elevator in a fire. Show your family where the stairs are located and practice using them. Make sure no stairways are blocked or locked.
• Stay low. Teach your children to avoid breathing in smoke and fumes, which tend to rise, and practice how to do this during your fire drill.
• Get out, then call. Don't waste precious time trying to reach the fire department. Call them after your family is safely out of the building.
• If you can't escape, seal yourself in. If both stairwells and hallway are filled with smoke, and you can't exit, seal your family in a room with a window using duct tape or towels around the door and over the air vents. Open the window to let in fresh air, but don't break it; you might need to close it if smoke comes in from outside the building.
• If you are trapped in the building, call the fire department to give them your exact location. Signal those at the scene by waving a flashlight or light-colored cloth.

dispatcher and those on the scene.

Be sure your street number is clearly visible. Can fire safety personnel clearly see your street number? You may need to add new numbering or paint the number onto the curb.

If you're trapped, seal out smoke. If your way out of the house is obstructed by fire, gather the family in one room and buy yourself some time by sealing out smoke. Seal the door frame and any vents with duct tape or towels. Then open the top and bottom of a window, if possible, and stand by it. Call the fire department with your exact location and wave a flashlight or a light-colored cloth so firefighters can see you. Teach this procedure to older children in case they get trapped alone.

Install smoke detectors on each level of your house. Put them outside sleeping areas, in bedrooms, the main living area, and the basement.

Keep fire extinguishers in strategic places. At a minimum, you should keep one on each floor and in the kitchen. Be sure you know how to use them. The one in the kitchen should be a multipurpose fire extinguisher, one that can put out electrical and grease fires. (See "Putting Out a Pan Fire," page 33.)

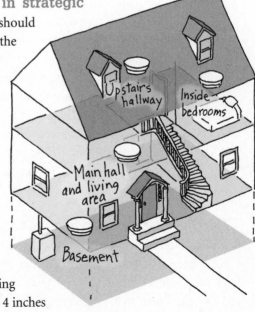

Install multiple smoke detectors in your home. If you have multiple levels, install a smoke detector up high on each level and outside sleeping areas. Mount each alarm at least 4 inches from a corner and 4 inches from walls, but away from windows and heating vents. It's best to install one inside each bedroom as well, especially because you and your children should sleep with bedroom doors closed.

Test your smoke detectors and replace the batteries. Test them every month and replace the batteries at least once a year. (A chirping sound means your battery needs to be replaced.) Pick the same dates every year to help you remember to change the batteries, for example, when you adjust the clocks for daylight saving time.

Never disable your smoke detector. Perhaps your smoke detector occasionally goes off while you are cooking. It's tempting to shut the thing off or remove the batteries. Never do this; you may forget to reset the detector or reinstall the batteries.

Install carbon monoxide detectors. Carbon monoxide is a byproduct of fuel combustion, present wherever fuel is burned. Typical sources are gas-fired appliances, including dryers and furnaces, wood-burning furnaces or fireplaces, and motor vehicles. Carbon monoxide poisoning often occurs when people are asleep; because of the colorless and odorless nature of the gas, many people don't realize they are being poisoned. That makes it crucial to install carbon monoxide detectors outside bedroom areas and on each level of your home. They should be able to detect both low and high concentrations of carbon monoxide because low concentrations over a long period of time are just as dangerous as high exposures over a short period. Proper placement is essential for these detectors to work, so be sure to read the owner's manual before you install them.

Maintain your carbon monoxide detectors. When you change the batteries on your smoke detectors, change them on your carbon monoxide detectors as well. Carbon monoxide detectors should last five years, so check the label on the bottom of detectors and replace any that are older than that.

Use Portable Electric Heaters Safely

Portable electrical heaters provide heat quickly and without the risk of carbon monoxide poisoning, making them a popular way to provide extra warmth to a chilly room. Of course, you'll want to keep your children away from space heaters—electrical or otherwise. Here are additional tips for safe use of portable electrical heaters:

• Keep portable heaters at least 3 feet away from upholstered furniture, drapes, bedding, and other combustible materials. Do not place heaters where towels, clothing, or the like could fall on the appliance and catch fire.

• Do not permit children to move the heater or adjust the controls.

• Avoid using an extension cord unless absolutely necessary. If you must use an extension cord, don't use a light-gauge household one. Use a heavy-gauge cord marked #14 AWG (American Wire Gauge) or #12 AWG. (The smaller the AWG number the greater the thickness of the wire.) Do not bury the cord under carpeting or rugs. Keep the cord stretched out—heat will build up in a coiled cord, possibly melting the insulation and causing a fire. Do not place anything on top of the cord. Only use extension cords bearing the label of an independent testing laboratory such as Underwriter's Laboratories (UL) or Electrical Testing Laboratories (ETL).

• Use the heater on the floor. Never place heaters on cabinets, tables or other furniture, or the like.

• Never use heaters for drying anything, including apparel or shoes.

• Turn off the heater when family members leave the house or are sleeping.

• Use a space heater that has been certified by a recognized testing laboratory.

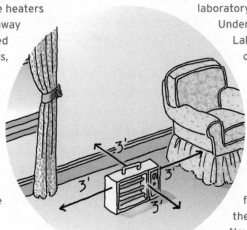

Keep space heaters at least 3 feet away from furniture, drapes and any other combustible materials.

Know carbon monoxide poisoning symptoms. At lower levels of exposure, carbon monoxide poisoning can be mistaken for the flu. The symptoms include dizziness, fatigue, headaches, nausea, and irregular breathing. But some people have no symptoms—another reason detectors are important. If you have any doubt about whether you have the flu or carbon monoxide poisoning, you should evacuate your home, call your local emergency number and stay away from your house until someone from the fire department says it's safe to return to your home.

Check heating appliances for leaks. A faulty furnace or fuel-burning heater can result in a carbon monoxide leak. You should have a professional service person inspect all your heating appliances, including their mechanical components, thermostat controls, and automatic safety devices, every year.

Be sure nothing is blocking your chimney or flue. A blocked chimney or flue can result in carbon monoxide gas becoming trapped. Rather than escaping and exiting the house through the chimney, this deadly gas can go back inside your house. Also, the cause of a blocked chimney is likely to be a build-up of creosote, which can cause a chimney fire. Be sure the flue is open and that neither the flue nor chimney have anything blocking it.

Use portable generators with caution. Beware of the possibility of carbon monoxide poisoning from the engine exhaust as well as the possibilities of electric shock, electrocution, fire, and burns. Carbon monoxide can build up within minutes when a generator is used in a confined or partly enclosed space. Never use one inside your home, garage, crawl space, shed, or similar area—even if you try to ventilate the space by using a fan or opening windows or doors.

Never use an oven or range as a source of heat. A gas oven may go out or not burn well, leading to carbon monoxide poisoning, and an electric oven or range could overheat. Besides, it's dangerous to children to leave an operating oven open or the burners on.

Make your kitchen safe. Cooking equipment is associated with more than 100,000 residential fires a year. Here are some tips to keep your family safe:

* Never place or store items that can be ignited near the range, including potholders, plastic utensils, towels, and other non-cooking equipment.
* Be careful of long sleeves and loose material. They can catch fire or become entangled with a pot handle, causing the pot to overturn. Roll up or fasten long sleeves with pins or elastic bands while cooking, or wear short sleeves or sleeves that fit your arms snugly.
* Do not reach across a range while cooking.
* Keep the storage area above the stove free of flammable and combustible items, including matches.
* Items that attract children (like cookies and candy) should not be kept above the range. They should be kept out of the immediate area.
* Don't leave the stove unattended when cooking.

Store flammable liquids outside the house. They have contributed to countless house fires. Be sure they are out of your children's reach and are in properly labeled, tightly closed, nonglass containers. Keep them away from heaters, water heaters, furnaces, ranges, and other electric and gas appliances.

Ban matches and lighters. Children playing with fire are the leading cause of child fire casualties, according to the U.S. Fire Administration. In fact, more than a third of the fires that kill children are set by children playing with fire. Children as young as 2 are capable of lighting matches and lighters, so they should always be kept out of your child's reach. Let your children know that matches are never to be touched or played with. Never use them to entertain your children.

Buy appropriate sleepwear for your child. It should be tight-fitting and/or flame-resistant. Your children may want to wear T-shirts to bed, but don't let them sleep in any loose-fitting or oversized garments made from fabrics that aren't flame-resistant.

Post emergency numbers. Keep the emergency phone number for the fire department, the police, etc. by each phone and make sure your children know how to call 911.

CHAPTER 17

Keeping
the
Lead Out

reventing exposure to lead is one of the most
important steps you can take to safeguard your child's
health. Breathing in or swallowing lead-contaminated dust, paint, or water can cause health problems for
people of any age, but lead is particularly dangerous for
young children, whose developing brains are especially vulnerable. They are also more likely to get this potent toxin
into their bodies because they frequently place their fingers, toys, and other potentially contaminated objects in
their mouths, and they absorb a greater proportion of
ingested lead than adults do. This chapter begins by out-
lining the problem, and then tells you what you can do to
prevent exposure.

Severe lead poisoning can cause seizures, coma and death, as illustrated by the 2006 death of a 4-year-old Minnesota boy who swallowed a lead-laden charm that came with a pair of Reebok shoes. Lower levels of lead poisoning can occur with no obvious symptoms. It frequently goes unrecognized, even though it can eventually cause lowered IQ, learning disabilities, and behavioral problems. Since there is no "safe" dose of lead, understanding its risks and doing everything you can to avoid exposure to this toxin is crucial.

While recalls of lead-tainted toys make headlines all too frequently, Americans' exposure to lead over much of the past century was driven by its industrial use and by two products in particular: paint and gasoline. For decades, lead was used as a pigment in paint and as an additive in gasoline. By the late 1980s, those two industries had each used about 6 million tons of the metal in the U.S., and the toxic residue still lingers.

Even though the federal government banned lead in gasoline and paint beginning in the 1970s, it is estimated that more than a third of the nation's housing stock still contains some lead paint and one out of four homes has significant lead-paint hazards. These hazards can include deteriorating lead paint, lead dust inside the home and lead in the soil around the foundation.

Drinking water can also be tainted by lead that leaches from older pipes and solder.

Among other sources of lead exposure are imported or antique toys made with lead paint, plastic products (including some vinyl baby bibs) that use lead as a stabilizer, and imported jewelry that appears to have been manufactured from electronic waste. Adults who have contact with lead either on the job, such as contractors renovating older homes, or through hobbies—spending time at an indoor firing range or in craft activities such as making pottery or stained glass—may in turn expose their families to it by wearing contaminated clothing.

Having Your Child Tested

Your pediatrician can do a simple blood test to assess the level of lead in your child's blood. The Environmental Protection Agency (EPA) recommends that all children have this test at age 1 and again at age 2. Some pediatricians also recommend testing at annual checkups for children under age 6, especially if they live in or frequently spend time in pre-1978 buildings.

Since the federal government banned lead in gasoline and house paint beginning in the 1970s, the average lead level in children under age 6 has dropped about 90 percent. The average for that age group in the U.S. in 2007 was slightly less than 2 micrograms of lead per deciliter of blood. Children whose levels are 10 micrograms or more are considered by the U.S. Centers for Disease Control (CDC) to be at increased risk for learning and behavioral problems.

But no "safe" blood lead level has been defined, and recent studies indicate that the greatest incremental damage to a child's brain appears to occur below the CDC's prevailing 10 micrograms standard, which was established in 1991. For instance, two thirds of the typical nine-point decline in IQ experienced by children with levels of lead between 10 and 30 micrograms might actually occur at levels below 10 micrograms, according to a July 2005 study by an international group of researchers. A growing number of scientists and public health officials therefore argue that the CDC should change its official definition of an elevated blood lead level to 5 micrograms per deciliter to reflect this new evidence about the harmful effects of low lead levels.

Be sure to ask your doctor for the specific numerical blood lead test results for your child because some pediatricians still simply report to parents that their children's levels are "normal" as long as they are below the CDC's 10-microgram standard. Knowing that your child's level is even slightly elevated should not be a cause for panic, but it can prompt you to search for and eliminate the sources of exposure.

Eliminating Lead Sources

Although lead levels peak in the toddler years when children are exploring their world with their mouths and hands, negative health effects are actually associated with lead exposure at any age, so it's wise to avoid contact with the substance no matter how old you are.

Also be aware that lead exposure can hurt your chances of having a baby because high levels can cause decreased fertility in men and also increase the odds of miscarriage in women. If you're pregnant, avoid areas where there is lead-based paint because you can pass the toxin to your fetus through your blood, potentially damaging your baby's developing brain. This is good advice for any woman of childbearing age, since lead stays in the body for a long time.

The following is a game plan to minimize lead risks for your family.

Cover bare soil. The major sources of lead exposure for children in the U.S. are deteriorating lead-based paint and lead-contaminated household dust or soil tracked into the home. Bare soil—which can be contaminated with residue from leaded-gasoline exhaust fumes as well as lead from paint or pesticides—should be covered by planting grass, piling mulch or wood chips on top of it, or by landscaping with sod or bushes.

The older your home, the more likely it is to pose lead-based paint risks. An estimated 68 percent of the homes built before 1940 contain lead paint, as well as 43 percent of those built from 1940 through 1959, and about 8 percent of those constructed from 1960 to 1977.

Helpful Booklets to Download

The EPA has published three booklets on lead exposure. One, called "Lead in Your Home: A Parent's Reference Guide," can be found at *www.epa.gov/lead/pubs/leadrev.pdf*. Another, "Protect Your Family from Lead in Your Home" can be downloaded at *www.epa.gov/lead/pubs/leadpdfe.pdf*. You may also want to download "Testing Your Home for Lead" at *www.epa.gov/lead/pubs/leadtest.pdf*.

Lead paint becomes a hazard when disturbed. All homes built before 1978 should be presumed to contain lead-based paint that may present a hazard unless a licensed lead inspector has determined otherwise. To find such an expert, or a licensed contractor for lead paint renovation work go to *www.epa.gov/lead/pubs/lead off1.htm*. Here you will find a listing of regional EPA offices. Call or send an e-mail message to your local office to obtain a list of EPA-certified lead-expert firms.

If paint on walls is not chipping or peeling, it's less likely to cause toxic exposure, but even intact paint can be a hazard, particularly on windows and doors that generate lead-contaminated dust when disturbed by impact or friction. Sanding or scraping releases large amounts of toxic lead dust, so renovations or repairs can be hazardous if performed improperly. For information on how to safely combat lead paint hazards, go to *www.hud.gov/offices/lead/healthyhomes/lead.cfm*.

Test your tap water. Lead can leach into drinking water from lead pipes, solder, brass fixtures or valves. If you are supplied by a public water system, your local water authority should provide data on whether its supply exceeds 15 parts per billion, the level at which the EPA requires water systems to begin controlling lead contamination. But the source of contamination could be in your home's plumbing rather than the public water supply, so testing water from your tap is the only way to know for sure whether it contains lead, since you can't see, taste or smell it. Call your local or state health department to find out how to test water in your home.

Replacing aging plumbing can eliminate the source of contamination, or you can install a filter certified to remove lead. In the meantime, you can reduce your risks by using only cold water for drinking or cooking. It's important to flush the tap by letting the cold water run for 12 minutes before using it, especially when the water has been off and sitting in the pipes for more than 12 hours. Lead-contaminated water poses particular risks for infants who drink formula made with tap water because of the large volume they consume relative to their body weight. The CDC recommends using only bottled water for formula preparation and for cooking and drinking if you are pregnant or have children in a home with water containing lead levels higher than the EPA's action level.

Identify and remove lead-tainted toys and other children's products. Start by checking *www.cpsc.gov* or *www.cdc.gov/nceh/lead/recalls* for photos and descriptions of toys, jewelry, and other products recalled because of lead-contamination. Follow manufacturers' instructions for returning recalled products.

Lead hazards are not limited to the millions of toys and jewelry items that have been recalled, however. Tests in CONSUMER REPORTS' labs have detected lead at varying levels in samples of toys, dishware, jewelry, glue stick caps, vinyl backpacks, children's ceramic tea sets and other items not included on any federal recall list. (See "Product Recalls," starting on page 194.)

Home testing kits find some lead. Some toys, including many imported from China, have been recalled because the paint used on them exceeded the U.S. Consumer Product Safety Commission's guidelines. Home lead-testing kits, such as Homax Lead Check, Lead Check Household Lead Test Kit, and Lead Inspector, can be useful though limited screening tools for detecting surface, or "accessible" lead. They don't, however, detect lead that may be embedded below the surface in items such as metal jewelry or plastic gluestick caps. While lead sealed below an item's surface may not transfer to children's hands and pose an immediate risk, experience with lead-tainted vinyl miniblinds in recent years suggests that exposure to sunlight and heat can cause some plastic items to release embedded lead over time as a product goes through normal wear and tear.

To determine exact lead levels, you would need to have items screened professionally, a process that's probably too expensive to do routinely for everyday items. If you are interested, the National Lead Information Center (800-424-LEAD) can provide a list of professionals who can test for lead using a variety of approved methods, including laboratory tests and inspections with a portable X-ray fluorescence (XRF) machines, which instantly assesses total lead content. As mentioned, you can also find professionals by contacting a local EPA office. You'll find this list at *www.epa.gov/lead/pubs/leadoff1.htm.*

Get in the Lead-Fighting Habit

Here are some day-to-day things you can do, along with some things to avoid, that can help to protect your family from lead exposure.

• Store toys in a clean place off the floor and wash them frequently to remove any accumulated dust or dirt that may contain lead.

• Sort through the toy box periodically to discard items with chipped paint, deteriorated plastic, or other broken or damaged parts.

• Avoid vintage toys and antique furniture that may have been painted with older lead-based paint. If an item is a keepsake or collectible, put it away until your child is older.

• Do not buy jewelry for young children. Not only have millions of pieces been recalled for excessive lead content, but such jewelry can also pose a choking hazard.

• Make sure arts and crafts items you buy for your children are nontoxic. Lead has been banned from paint, including children's paints, but artist's paints and ceramic glazes for adult use are exempt from the ban and can contain lead and other toxic heavy metals.

• Wrap all food that goes in your child's lunch box, including fruit. Certain vinyl lunch boxes have been found to contain lead.

• Although most large commercial producers of ceramic dishware meet regulatory standards for lead, not all do, especially overseas producers. Pottery that is homemade or purchased abroad at open markets or from street sellers, as well as small producers from other countries, may also pose risks, so avoid serving food in it.

• Don't allow babies to play with or chew on your keys because metal keys have been identified as potential sources of lead exposure.

• Garden hoses, extension or power cords and strands of holiday lights often contain lead (which may be disclosed on their labeling), so anyone handling them should wash their hands afterward.

• Vinyl miniblinds manufactured before 1996 may contain lead that forms dust on the blinds as the plastic deteriorates from sun and heat exposure. Remove them if you think they were manufactured before 1996.

• Feed your child a diet rich in iron and calcium. Children who consume adequate amounts of those nutrients absorb less lead.

• Check recall lists regularly in case any items in your home have been recalled due to excessive lead levels.

Product Recalls

Following is a list of recent recalls of some children's products from the Consumer Product Safety Commission. This is a sampling and does not include every product or product category. For more information about these recalls and additional recalls, go to *www.cpsc.gov*. CPSC also offers an email subscription list concerning any recalls of infant and child products. Sign up at *www.cpsc.gov/cpsclist.aspx*.

If you own a recalled product, CPSC advises that you stop using the product immediately unless otherwise instructed. In some cases, you may contact the manufacturer or retailer to receive a product replacement, replacement parts, a free repair kit, a refund or new instructions on how to use the product.

Always fill out and return any warrantee or registration card that comes with a product so the manufacturer can notify you in case of a recall. (Cards are required for child safety seats but are optional for other juvenile products.)

Child safety and booster seats are not included in the following list. These are under the jurisdiction of the National Highway Traffic Safety Administration. Recalls for both independent seats and integral child seats that are part of a vehicle can be found at *www-odi .nhtsa.dot.gov/cars/problems/recalls/childseat.cfm*. The site also offers a child safety seat registration form you can fill out that NHTSA will forward to the manufacturer.

Report any unsafe product at *www.cpsc.gov* or call 800-638-2772. You'll find a form to report a child safety seat problem at the NHTSA Web site above. Or you can call 888-327-4236.

Arts and Crafts
Discount School Supply shaving paintbrushes
Spin Master Aqua Dots
J.C. Penney Deluxe wood art sets
Cracker Barrel Old Country Store Princess
Magnetic travel art set lap desks
Discount School Supply children's Elite
5-in-1 easels
Target jumbo pencils with sharpeners
Bernat Yarn "Fur Out" yarn

Baby Feeding Items
Next Step Plastic sippy/tumbler cups
BabySwede LLC BabyBjorn feeding spoons

Baby Seats (nonbath)
RC2 The First Years newborn-to-toddler
reclining feeding seats
RC2 The First Years 3-in-1 Flush and Sounds
potty seats
Bumbo International Baby Sitter Seats

Baby Walkers and Stationary Entertainers
Ace Han baby walkers
Bike Pro Inc. baby walkers
SunTome baby walkers
Big Save International Corp. baby walkers
PlayKids USA baby walkers
Dream On Me Industries baby walkers
Graco Children's Products Bumble Bee toys
with blue antennae

Bathtubs and Seats (new instructions and parts)
Dorel Juvenile Group safety alert for 1st
Tubside bath seats
The First Years Inc. new safety instructions
for combo baby tubs/step stools
Gerry Baby Products Company Splash Seats
replacement suction cups

Bouncers and Jumpers
Oeuf LLC infant bouncer seats
Kids II Inc. Bounce Bounce Baby! doorway
jumpers
Kids II Inc. Bright Starts Jammin' doorway
jumpers

Bumper Pads
Pottery Barn Kids matelasse crib bumpers

Bunk Beds
Hooker Furniture bunk beds
d-Scan Jubee bunk beds
PJ Sleep Shop wooden twin/twin, twin/
double and loft bunk beds
Coaster Co. of America metal twin/twin and
twin/full bunk beds
Ashley Furniture Industries Inc. Trail's End,
Cottage Retreat and Stages bunk beds
Ethan Allen bunk beds

Changing Tables
Scandinavian Child Cariboo folding
changing tables
Childcraft Education wooden changing tables
with steps

Children's Clothing
Seventy Two Inc. Bonafide Love hooded
children's sweatshirts with hood drawstring

Gap Outlet Warmest Jacket boys' jackets with waist drawstring

Liberty Apparel Jewel girls' hooded sweatshirts with hood drawstring

Scope Apparel boys' hooded sweatshirts with hood drawstring

Sears Personal Identity V-neck sweaters with hood drawstring

Kmart Basic Editions girls' clothing sets with waist drawstring

TKS children's pants with ribbon belt

Old Navy performance-fleece-lined boys' jackets with waist drawstring toggle

Bon-Ton Department Stores Inc. children's fleece hooded zip-up jackets and bathrobes

Life is Good Inc. Zippity Hoodie and Sherpa full zip children's hooded sweatshirts with drawstrings

Paramount Apparel International toddler and youth nylon bucket hats

Kmart Basic Editions girls' clothing sets

Nordstrom Pine Peak Blues children's jackets

Creative Expressions children's party hats

Personalized Infant Red Baby long johns

Samara Brothers boys' three-piece short sets

Mervyns Little Girls Capri pants with snap roll cuff

Disney Store children's footed pajamas

Hanna Andersson children's crossover tee and lounge pants sets and cropped johns

Children's Furniture

Netshops children's table and chair sets

Jetmax International children's wooden storage rack

Hold Everything Homeroom Bedroom Collection plastic hardware covers on children's furniture

Summit Marketing International LLC children's folding chairs

Atico International USA children's folding chairs

Royal Seating Ltd. Prima Chair

Delta Enterprise Corp. director's chairs for children

Meco Corp. Kid's Essentials five-piece folding furniture sets red chair

Children's Jewelry

Codee International Corp. Codeena Princess children's metal jewelry

Raymond Geddes & Co. children's pencil pouches

Buy-Rite Sparkle City charm bracelets and tack pin sets

Colossal Jewelry & Accessories children's metal necklaces and bracelets

La Femme NY Inc. children's necklace and earring sets

Pure Allure Crystal Innovations jewelry (sold at Michaels stores)

Family Dollar Stores Rachel Rose and Distinctly Basics assorted metal jewelry

Exclusively at Limited Too Stores decorative packaging pearl-like bead attachments sold with girl's gift sets

Dollar Tree Stores Inc. Beary Cute, Expressions, and Sassy & Chic children's metal jewelry

WeGlow International children's metal jewelry

Rhode Island Novelty children's spinning wheel metal necklaces

Buy-Rite children's Divine Inspiration charm bracelets

Toby N.Y.C. Toby & Me jewelry sets

Uncas Manufacturing Co Sleeping Beauty Crown and Cinderella Star earring sets (sold at Wal-Mart Stores in Florida)

Future Industries Essentials for Kids jewelry sets

GeoCentral butterfly necklaces

Crimzon Rose Accessories silver stud earrings (sold exclusively at Kmart)

Tween Brands children's metal jewelry (sold at Limited Too and Justice Stores, Limited Too catalog and Web site)

Cardinal Distributing children's turquoise rings

Spandrel Sales and Marketing children's necklaces, bracelets and rings

Cardinal Distributing children's rings with dice or horseshoes

Oriental Trading Company Inc. children's religious fish necklaces

Cardinal Distributing Co. children's charm bracelets and Sportswear necklaces

A&A Global Industries children's Groovy Grabber bracelets

Cribs

Bassettbaby Wendy Bellissimo Collection convertible cribs (sold exclusively at Babies "R" Us)

Simplicity Inc. cribs

NettoCollection Moderne and Loft cribs

Stokke Sleepi crib foam mattresses

Song Lin Industrial Inc. sleigh round cribs

Simplicity Inc. Graco-branded Aspen cribs

Delta Enterprise Corp. Lov's Europa natural color cribs (sold exclusively at Toys "R" Us)

Child Craft Industries, Inc. cribs

Pottery Barn Kids spindle cribs

Delta Enterprise Corp. portable cribs

Orbelle Trade Inc. cribs

Games

Cranium Cadoo board games

Far East Brokers fishing games (sold at grocery stores)

SimplyFun Ribbit board games

Global Design Concepts magnetic game pieces sold with "Cars"-themed backpacks

Target Anima Bamboo Collection games

Nintendo of America replacement program for wrist straps used with controllers for the Wii video game system

Chicken Limbo electronic party games

Sony Computer Entertainment America Inc. certain AC adaptors sold with slim version PlayStation 2 Systems

Hidden Hills Productions, Inc. Maptangle World Edition floor mat games

High Chairs

Graco Children's Products Inc. Contempo high chairs

Pacifiers and Accessories

Shims Bargain Babytown pacifiers

Sailing (U.S.) International Corp. flashing pacifiers and 2-in-1 flashing pacifiers with whistle necklaces

Various firms' pacifiers decorated with crystals: Dara Linda's Baby Bling and Jewelry Design, Bling Toes, Baby Bling Things, PeaNaPod Bling and Accessories, MJM Crystal Designs

Various firms flashing pacifiers: Rhode Island Novelty, Hayes Specialties Corp., My Bargain Bin LLC, Ravesupply.com, Dollar Days International LLC

Kole Imports Baby 2-pack pacifiers

Ideal Distributors Inc. Cachito pacifiers

Delta Enterprise Corp. Lov's decorated orthodontic pacifiers

California International Trading light-up pacifier

Solar Inc. flashing toy pacifiers and 2-in-1

flashing pacifier with whistle necklace

The Elegant Kids 2000 Inc. Soother
baby pacifiers

Todo Dollar Wholesale flashing pacifiers with
whistle necklace and flashing pacifiers shock
baby necklace

Play Yards

Kolcraft play yards sold under Kolcraft
Travelin' Tot, Carter's Lennon Travelin' Tot,
Sesame Beginnings, Jeep Sahara and Contours
3-in-1 labels

Rattles

Target Plush Boys and Plush Baby rattles

Tri-Star International ball rattles and
whistle rattles

Tiffany & Co. Paloma rattles and Farm
Teether rattles

Sippy and Tumbler Cups

Starbucks children's plastic cups

Dollar General Frankenstein tumblers

CVS/pharmacy Playskool sippy cups

Strollers and Accessories

Stokke Xplory strollers (serial numbers 1
through 27,295 and 27,698 through 28,097)

Regal Lager Inc. Phil & Teds e3 strollers with
double seats and twin buggy

Sycamore Kids Inc. Mountain Buggy
Urban Single and Urban Double, and Breeze
jogging strollers

Kelty Speedster, Speedster Deluxe and
Speedster Deuce jogging strollers

Graco Children's Products Inc. Duo Tandem
and certain MetroLite strollers

Swings

Fisher-Price Rainforest open top take-along
infant swings

Graco Children's Products Travel Lite swings

Teething Items

Elegant Baby heart and car sterling silver
teethers

Empire Silver sterling silver teething rings

Infantino Lion teethers

Priddy Trucks shaker teether books

Kids II Inc. Bright Starts Star and Bright
Starts teether beads

Prestige Toy Corp. Spinning Water teethers

Toy Animals

Victoria's Secret holiday cosmetics stuffer
bears (sold exclusively at store's Web site)

Schylling Associates Duck Family collectable
wind-up toys

The Orvis Company stuffed plush horse
pillows and fairy dolls (sold with sleeping bags)

Tri-Star International wind-up toys

Fisher-Price Laugh and Learn bunny toys

Wal-Mart Holiday Time stuffed Christmas
beagles and baby Cookie Monster toys

Fun Express bendable dog and cat toys (given
away at libraries)

The Little Tikes Co. Glowin' Dino and
Glowin' Doggy animal-shaped flashlights
(sold at Target)

Douglas Company Sparkle Horse plush toys

Pokémon USA Pokémon plush toys

Ocean Desert Sales Inc. stuffed yarn bunnies

Toys

West Music egg-shaker toy instruments

Sears and Kmart My First Kenmore play stoves

AAFES Soldier Bear toys

Dollar Tree Stores Baby Toys bead and wire toys and Speed Racer Pull Back & Go Action! cars

Paricon Children's Snow and Sand Castle kits (sold exclusively at LL Bean)

Schylling Associates Robot 2000 collectable tin robot, Dizzy Ducks music boxes, Winnie-the-Pooh spinning tops, and Thomas and Friends, Curious George and other spinning tops and tin Pails

Fisher-Price Laugh & Learn kitchen toys

The Gymboree Corp. toy pirate swords

Dunkin' Donuts pink and orange glow sticks (free giveaway with donuts)

Kipp Brothers bendable dinosaur toys

CKI children's decorating sets (sold exclusively at Toys "R" Us)

Eveready Battery Co. "Pirates of the Caribbean" medallion squeeze-toy flashlights

KB Toys wooden pull-along alphabet and math blocks wagons, wooden pull-along learning blocks wagons, 10-in-1 activity learning carts, and flip-flop alphabet books

RC2 Knights of the Sword series toys

Fisher-Price Big Big World 6-in-1 bongo band toys, and Sesame Street, Dora the Explorer and other licensed character toys

Easy Bake, a division of Hasbro, Inc., Easy-Bake ovens

Target Play Wonder toy barbeque grills

Gemmy Industries Corp. flashing eyeball toys

Small World Toys IQ Preschool take-apart townhouses

Mega Brands Magnetix Magnetic building set

Geometix International LLC MagneBlocks magnetic construction toys

RC2 toy keys

Alex Super cooking sets

RadioShack Corp. Child Guidance toy pliers

BRIO Corp. pull-along snail

Toy Chests and Trunks

Delta Enterprise Corp. Cars toy storage benches (sold exclusively at Toys "R" Us)

Stork Craft Manufacturing Inc. Stork Craft toy boxes

Pottery Barn Kids Cameron toy chests

Toy Play Sets and Activity Sets

Battat Magnabild magnetic building systems

Toys "R" Us Elite Operations Super Rigs, Command Patrol Center, Barracuda Helicopter and 3-pack, 8-inch figures

J.C. Penney Disney Winnie-the-Pooh play sets

Mattel Barbie accessory toys, Polly Pocket dolls and accessories, Doggie Day Care magnetic toys, Barbie and Tanner play sets with magnets

Kipp Brothers Mag Stix magnetic building sets

Graco Children's Products Soft Blocks Tower Toys on Graco Baby Einstein Discover and Play activity centers

Target Little Tree Wood activity cart toys

Toys "R" Us Elite Operations toy sets